Biology of the Neonate

Foetal and Neonatal Research

Founded 1959 as 'Biologia Neonatorum' by A. Minkowski
(formerly 'Etudes Néo-Natales')

KARGER

Printed in Switzerland
on acid-free paper by
Thür AG Offsetdruck, Pratteln

Appears monthly:
2 volumes per year (12 issues)

Biology of the Neonate

Submission: Only original papers written in English are considered and should be sent to:

S. Karger AG
Editorial Dept. 'Biology of the Neonate'
P.O. Box
CH–4009 Basel (Switzerland)

Manuscripts should be submitted in triplicate (with three sets of illustrations of which one is an original), typewritten double-spaced on one side of the paper, with a wide margin.

Conditions: All manuscripts are subject to editorial review. Manuscripts are received with the explicit understanding that they are not under simultaneous consideration by any other publication. Submission of an article for publication implies the transfer of the copyright from the author to the publisher upon acceptance. Accepted papers become the permanent property of 'Biology of the Neonate' and may not be reproduced by any means, in whole or in part, without the written consent of the publisher. It is the author's responsibility to obtain permission to reproduce illustrations, tables, etc. from other publications.

Brief communications: Short reports, including case reports, brief laboratory observations, and preliminary communications, may be submitted for accelerated publication under 'brief communications'. To qualify for rapid publication, such reports should not exceed a printed length of two pages, i.e., generally not more than 1,000 words of text accompanied by 2 figures or tables and from 5 to 10 references.

Arrangement

Title page: The first page of each paper should indicate the title (main title underlined), the authors' names, and the institute where the work was conducted. A short title for use as running head as well as the full address of the author to whom correspondence should be sent are also required.

Key words: For indexing purposes, a list of 3–10 key words in English is essential.

Abstract: Each paper needs an abstract of up to 10 lines.

Small type: Paragraphs which can or must be set in smaller type (case histories, test methods, etc.) should be indicated with a 'p' (petit) in the margin on the left-hand side.

Footnotes: Avoid footnotes. When essential, they are numbered consecutively and typed at the foot of the appropriate page.

Tables and illustrations: Tables and illustrations (both numbered in Arabic numerals) should be prepared on separate sheets. Tables require a heading and figures a legend, also prepared on a separate sheet. For the reproduction of illustrations, only good drawings and original photographs can be accepted; negatives or photocopies cannot be used. When possible, group several illustrations on one block for reproduction (max. size 144 × 196 mm) or provide crop marks. On the back of each illustration, indicate its number, the author's name, and 'top'. Color illustrations are reproduced at the author's expense.

References: In the text identify references by Arabic numerals [in square brackets]. Material submitted for publication but not yet accepted should be noted as 'unpublished data' and not be included in the reference list. The list of references should include only those publications which are cited in the text. Do not alphabetize; number references in the order in which they are first mentioned in the text. The surnames of the authors followed by initials should be given. There should be no punctuation other than a comma to separate the authors. Cite all authors, 'et al' is not sufficient. Abbreviate journal names according to the Index Medicus system. (Also see International Committee of Medical Journal Editors: Uniform requirements for manuscripts submitted to biomedical journals. Br Med J 1988;296:401–405.)

Examples

(a) Papers published in periodicals: Kauffman HF, van der Heide S, Beaumont F, Blok H, de Vries K: Class-specific antibody determination against *Aspergillus fumigatus* by means of the enzyme-linked immunosorbent assay. III. Comparative study: IgG, IgA, IgM ELISA titers, precipitating antibodies and IgE binding after fractionation of the antigen. Int Arch Allergy Appl Immunol 1986;80:300–306.

(b) Monographs: Matthews DE, Farewell VT: Using and Understanding Medical Statistics. Basel, Karger, 1985.

(c) Edited books: Hardy WD Jr, Essex M: FeLV-induced feline acquired immune deficiency syndrome: A model for human AIDS; in Klein E (ed): Acquired Immunodeficiency Syndrome. Prog Allergy. Basel, Karger, 1986, vol 37, pp 353–376.

Full address: The exact postal address complete with postal code must be given at the bottom of the title page. Please supply also Phone and Fax numbers.

Further details: Authors may consult our leaflet 'Rules for the Preparation of Manuscripts', available on request from the Publisher, S. Karger AG, P.O. Box, CH–4009 Basel (Switzerland).

Page charges: There is no page charge for papers of 6 or fewer printed pages (including tables, illustrations and references). Each additional complete or partial page is charged to the author at SFr. 225.– / US $ 150.00. The allotted size of a paper is equal to approx. 12 manuscript pages (including tables, illustrations and references).

Galley proofs: Unless indicated otherwise, galley proofs are sent to the first-named author and should be returned with the least possible delay. Alterations made in galley proofs, other than the correction of printer's errors, are charged to the author. No page proofs are supplied.

Reprints: Order forms and a price list are sent with the galley proofs. Orders submitted after the issue is printed are subject to considerably higher prices. Allow five weeks from date of publication for delivery of reprints.

KARGER

General Information

Biology of the Neonate

Publication data: 'Biology of the Neonate' is published 12 times annually. Volumes 61–62 with 6 issues each appear in 1992.
Subscription rates: Subscriptions run for a full calendar year. Prices are given per volume, surface postage included.
Personal subscription:
SFr. 307.30, US$ 205.10.
(Must be in the name of, billed to, and paid by an individual. Order must be marked 'personal subscription'.)
Institutional subscription:
(Regular rate.) SFr. 439.–, US$ 293.00.
Members of The Neonatal Society; Société Française de Néonatologie:
SFr. 131.70, US$ 87.90.
Airmail postage: SFr. 35.–, US$ 25.00.
(Extra per volume.)
Microform subscription:
SFr. 219.50, US$ 146.50.
(Available exclusively to subscribers of the paper edition.)
Single issues and back volumes: Information on availability and prices can be obtained through the Publisher.
Advertising: Correspondence and rate requests should be addressed to the Publisher.

Subscription orders: Orders can be placed at agencies, bookstores, directly with the Publisher S. Karger AG, P.O. Box, CH – 4009 Basel (Switzerland)
or with any of the following distributors:
Deutschland, Österreich, Ost-Europa:
S. Karger GmbH, Lörracher Strasse 16A
Postfach, D-W-7800 Freiburg
France: Librairie Luginbühl
36, bd de Latour-Maubourg, F-75007 Paris
Great Britain, Ireland:
S. Karger Publishers
11 Ravenscroft Road
Beckenham, Kent BR3 4TP
USA: S. Karger Publishers, Inc.
26 West Avon Road, P.O. Box 529
Farmington, CT 06085
India, Bangladesh, Sri Lanka:
S. Karger India Subscription Agency
B – 5/132 Safdarjung Enclave
New Delhi-110029
Japan: Katakura Libri, Inc.
36-9 Hongo 3-chome, Bunkyo-ku
Tokyo 113
Change of address: Both old and new address should be stated and sent to the subscription source.

Bibliographic indices: This journal is regularly listed in bibliographic services, including *Current Contents®*.
Book Reviews: Books are accepted for review by special agreement.
Copying: This journal has been registered with the Copyright Clearance Center (CCC), as indicated by the code appearing on the first page of each article. For readers in the US, this code signals consent for copying of articles for personal or internal use, or for the personal or internal use of specific clients, provided that the stated fee is paid per copy directly to CCC, 21 Congress Street, Salem, MA 01970 (USA). A copy of the first page of the article must accompany payment. Consent does not extend to copying for general distribution, for promotion, for creating new works, or for resale. In these cases, specific written permission must be obtained from the copyright owner, S. Karger AG, P.O. Box, CH – 4009 Basel (Switzerland).

KARGER

Editors:
Yukio Fukuyama,
Yoshiyuki Suzuki,
Shigehiko Kamoshita,
Paul Casaer

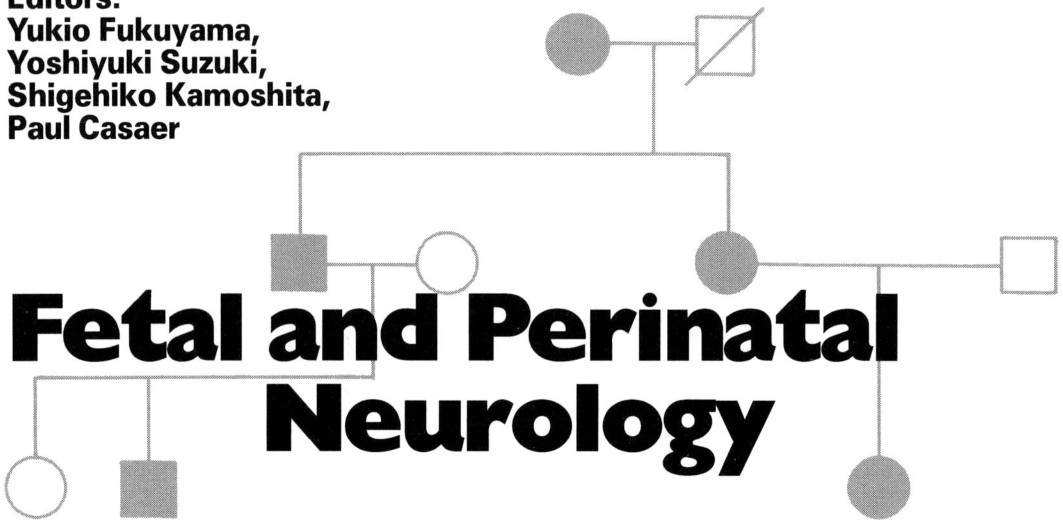

Fetal and Perinatal Neurology

This timely volume offers a broad survey of current research in fetal and perinatal neurology and assesses the most recent developments in the diagnosis and therapy of problematic neurological disorders. Recorded from an international symposium, the authoritative contributions feature up-to-date information on a wide spectrum of topical subjects from the application of advances in molecular genetics to ethical issues in child neurology. Two special award lectures review autism as a syndrome of neurological dysfunction and the physiological and pathophysiological roles of excitatory amino acids during central nervous system development. Providing convenient access to important international investigations, this book serves as a valuable guide to progress being made in both general areas and specific problems as well as to future research directions. It is an excellent resource for researchers in neurology and for clinicians concerned with the management and prevention of neurological disorders.

Fields of Interest

Neurology; Pediatrics; Embryology, Genetics, Metabolism, Molecular Biology, Pathology, Perinatal Medicine, Physiology

Main Headings

Award Lectures
Rapin, I.: Autism: A Syndrome of Neurological Dysfunction. Frank Ford Memorial Lecture 1990 · Johnston, M.V.: Physiological and Pathophysiological Roles of Excitatory Amino Acids during Central Nervous System Development. John Prichard Award Lecture 1990

Pediatric Neurogenetics

Embryology and Dysgenesis of the Brain

Neurocutaneous Syndromes

Pre- and Perinatal Pathophysiology of Brain Damage

New Syndromes and Rare Interesting Diseases in Child Neurology

Ethical Problems in Child Neurology

Fetal and Perinatal Neurology
Joint Convention of the 5th International Child Neurology Congress and the 3rd Asian and Oceanian Congress of Child Neurology, Tokyo, November 1990
Editors: Fukuyama, Y.; Suzuki, Y.; Kamoshita, S. (Tokyo); Casaer, P. (Leuven)
VIII + 388 p., 84 fig., 62 tab., hard cover, 1992
SFr. 290.– / DM 347.– / £ 126.10 / US$ 232.00
US$ price for USA, £ price for UK only (subject to change)
ISBN 3-8055-5398-6

KI 92515

KARGER

Experimental and Clinical Aspects of Surfactant Replacement

Experimental and Clinical Aspects of Surfactant Replacement

Selected papers from the 6th European Workshop on Surfactant Replacement, Héviz, Hungary, May 10–12, 1991

Guest Editors
Bengt Robertson, Stockholm
Henry L. Halliday, Belfast
Christian P. Speer, Göttingen
Béla Büky, Budapest

24 figures and 12 tables, 1992

KARGER

Biology of the Neonate

Vol. 61, Supplement 1, 1992

S. Karger
Medical and Scientific Publishers
Basel · München · Paris · London
New York · New Delhi · Bangkok
Singapore · Tokyo · Sydney

Drug Dosage
The authors and the publisher have exerted every effort to ensure that drug selection and dosage set forth in this text are in accord with current recommendations and practice at the time of publication. However, in view of ongoing research, changes in government regulations, and the constant flow of information relating to drug therapy and drug reactions, the reader is urged to check the package insert for each drug for any change in indications and dosage and for added warnings and precautions. This is particularly important when the recommended agent is a new and/or infrequently employed drug.

Printed in Switzerland on acid-free paper by
Thür AG Offsetdruck, Pratteln
ISBN 3-8055-5644-6

Contents

Biol Neonate 1992;61(suppl 1):1

Preface

Bengt Robertson, Stockholm
Henry L. Halliday, Belfast
Christian P. Speer, Göttingen
Béla Büky, Budapest

Surfactant replacement is now an established treatment for neonatal respiratory distress syndrome (RDS), reducing both incidence of complications and mortality. One of the first large randomized trials documenting these effects was reported by the Collaborative European Multicenter Study Group [Pediatrics 1988;88:683–691] and since then this group has continued to coordinate clinical and experimental work related to surfactant replacement therapy and to arrange annual meetings. The present supplement is based on 10 selected presentations from the 6th annual meeting held in Héviz, Hungary, May 10–11, 1991. These contributions deal with a wide range of topics, including biological significance of antibodies to surfactant proteins, computer-aided analysis of bubble stability for evaluation of surfactant function, experience from new clinical trials of surfactant replacement, effects of surfactant treatment on cerebral blood flow, airway phospholipid profile and lung mechanics, incidence of retinopathy in surfactant-treated babies, and costs of surfactant treatment for prophylaxis and treatment of neonatal RDS. Although most of the information contained in the papers relate to one particular surfactant preparation, Curosurf®, we feel that the results and ideas presented in the supplement should be of interest to many basic investigators in the field as well as to neonatologists who have adopted, or plan to adopt, this new therapeutic approach in their hospitals. We are grateful to the Chief Editor of *Biology of the Neonate* for this opportunity to introduce the activity of the Collaborative European Multicenter Study Group to a large circle of readers.

Original Paper

Biol Neonate 1992;61(suppl 1):2–14

David S. Strayer

Department of Pathology and Cell Biology, Thomas Jefferson University, Philadelphia, Pa., USA

Applications of Anti-Curosurf Antibodies to Understanding the Biology of Alveolar Surfactant

Key Words
Pulmonary surfactants
Antibodies, anti-idiotypic
Antibodies, monoclonal
Membrane proteins
Surfactant protein A

Abstract
The structure of surfactant-binding proteins from alveolar cell membranes was investigated using monoclonal anti-idiotypic antibodies directed against surfactant-binding regions of anti-surfactant monoclonal antibodies. Two different series of monoclonal anti-surfactant antibodies were used. One series included antibodies against rabbit surfactant, and the other antibodies against porcine surfactant. In addition, two monoclonal anti-idiotype antibodies were made. These anti-idiotype antibodies, called A2R and A2C, bind both anti-Curosurf and anti-rabbit surfactant antibodies comparably. They recognize a 30-kDa cell membrane protein on alveolar and bronchial epithelial cells. In addition, A2C and A2R block the binding of radiolabeled surfactant to these cells. Using a combination of A2C and A2R cDNA expression libraries from both human and porcine lungs were screened. One independent clone was identified in each library that produced protein that bound these monoclonal antibodies. The protein encoded by the cDNA in each clone bound radiolabeled recombinant surfactant protein-A. It is concluded that human and porcine alveolar cell SP-A binding proteins have been identified and its cDNA cloned. The potential implications of this finding for the understanding and treatment of surfactant deficiency states are considerable.

Introduction

Pulmonary surfactant is a complex mixture of proteins and phospholipids. The protein constituents of surfactant include protein A (SP-A), an apoprotein of 30–35 kDa, with the variability reflecting differing degrees of glycosylation. In its secreted form, SP-A is glycosylated [1]. SP-B, an 8–10 kDa protein, is far more hydrophobic, and occurs

David S. Strayer, PhD, MD
Department of Pathology and Cell Biology
Thomas Jefferson University
1020 Locust Street
Philadelphia, PA 19107 (USA)

in the lung mainly as a homodimer of approximately 18 kDa [2]. The smallest surfactant protein is SP-C, a 3.5-kDa protein that is among the most hydrophobic proteins known [3]. A fourth surfactant-associated protein of 39–43 kDa, SP-D, has recently been described, and partially characterized structurally, and its cDNA has been cloned [4].

The functions of these surfactant proteins are not completely understood. Thus, SP-A appears to stabilize tertiary and quaternary surfactant structures in vivo and in vitro. There is also evidence to suggest that it may protect surfactant mixtures from inhibition by other proteins [5]. In addition, it may play a role in inflammatory processes and phagocytic activities in the lung. Its role in lowering surface tension is not clear, SP-B, however, appears to be the principal protein constituent of surfactant mixtures that mediates surfactant's ability to lower surface tension [2]. The function of SP-C is not established. In some preparations, SP-C appears to be important in reducing surface tension [6]. Whether SP-C or SP-B is 'the' principal protein constituent of surfactant that determines its ability to lower surface tension in vitro is not known, and the roles of these two proteins in vivo are even less clear. The function of SP-D remains to be described.

These proteins, together with phospholipids, are secreted from alveolar type II pneumocytes and form the air-liquid interphase in the alveoli. The means by which this secretory process is regulated are beginning to be understood. SP-A, which is both secreted and recycled by type II cells, is probably very important in modulating phospholipid secretion by type II cells. Recent work indicates that SP-A binds to type II cells via a high-affinity specific receptor and that SP-A binding to its receptor down-regulates the production of surfactant from type II cells [7–9].

To date, little is known about the structure of this receptor. Clearly, in its ability to regulate the production of surfactant, it is a critical part of surfactant homeostasis. Perhaps an understanding of this receptor's function and structure may permit manipulation of surfactant secretion both in physiologic states and in pathologic states when insufficient surfactant is produced (neonatal respiratory distress syndrome; RDS), when surfactant is present in normal amounts but is abnormally inhibited by other proteins (adult RDS), or when surfactant is produced in abnormally large quantities (alveolar proteinosis). With these ends in mind, studies were performed to determine the structure of the receptor for surfactant on alveolar lining cells.

Experimental Approach

The approach to identifying a surfactant receptor is illustrated in figure 1. Since there was insufficient receptor protein to raise antibodies or to sequence directly, anti-receptor antibody was produced utilizing the principle of molecular mimicry. It was assumed that as anti-surfactant antibody binds to surfactant and as surfactant receptor also binds to surfactant, these two binding structures should resemble each other in their ligand recognition sites. Thus, antibody directed against the idiotypic, or antigen-binding, sites of anti-surfactant antibody might recognize the binding site on the surfactant receptor. In so doing, this anti-idiotype antibody should be able to displace surfactant from its receptor.

In principle, an anti-idiotypic antibody that can both bind surfactant receptor and inhibit surfactant-cell interactions could be used to screen cDNA expression libraries, identify cDNA encoding the surfactant recep-

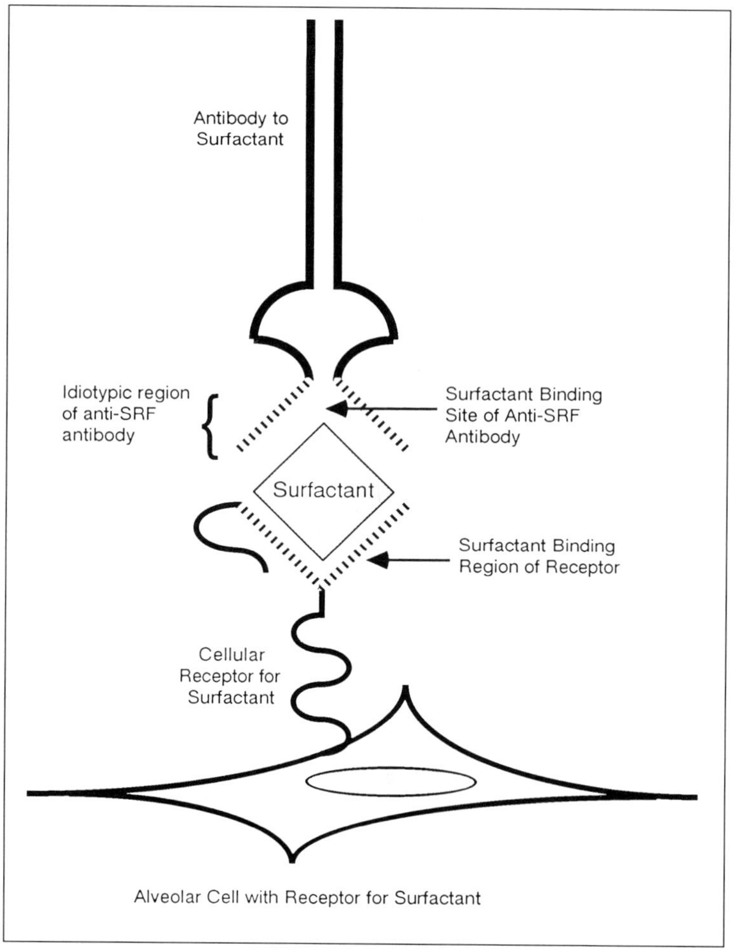

a

Fig. 1. Generation of antibody to surfactant receptor protein. In theory, if two molecules bind the same ligand, the ligand-binding sites of these two molecules should be similar. Surfactant protein bound by the specific receptor on cell membranes should thus share with anti-surfactant antibodies (anti-SRF) a common surfactant-binding region. Antibodies directed to the anti-surfactant antibodies might, therefore, recognize the surfactant-binding site of the surfactant receptor. In so doing, it would be expected that they would be able to displace surfactant protein from its receptor. This sequence of theoretical constructs as applied to the surfactant-surfactant receptor system is illustrated in these three panels. **a** Surfactant-binding sites on anti-surfactant antibody and surfactant receptor are similar. **b** Anti-idiotype antibody recognizes surfactant-binding site on anti-surfactant antibody and therefore has structure similar to that of surfactant itself. **c** Anti-(anti-surfactant) antibody recognizes the cell's surfactant receptor and blocks the interaction of this receptor with surfactant.

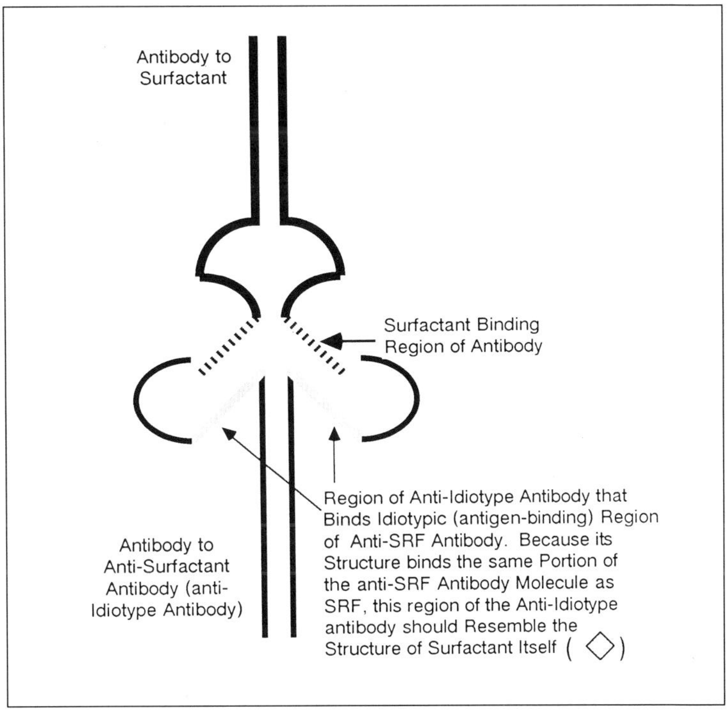
Antibody to
Surfactant
Surfactant Binding
Region of Antibody
Antibody to
Anti-Surfactant
Antibody (anti-
Idiotype Antibody)
Region of Anti-Idiotype Antibody that
Binds Idiotypic (antigen-binding) Region
of Anti-SRF Antibody. Because its
Structure binds the same Portion of
the anti-SRF Antibody Molecule as
SRF, this region of the Anti-Idiotype
antibody should Resemble the
Structure of Surfactant Itself (◇)

b

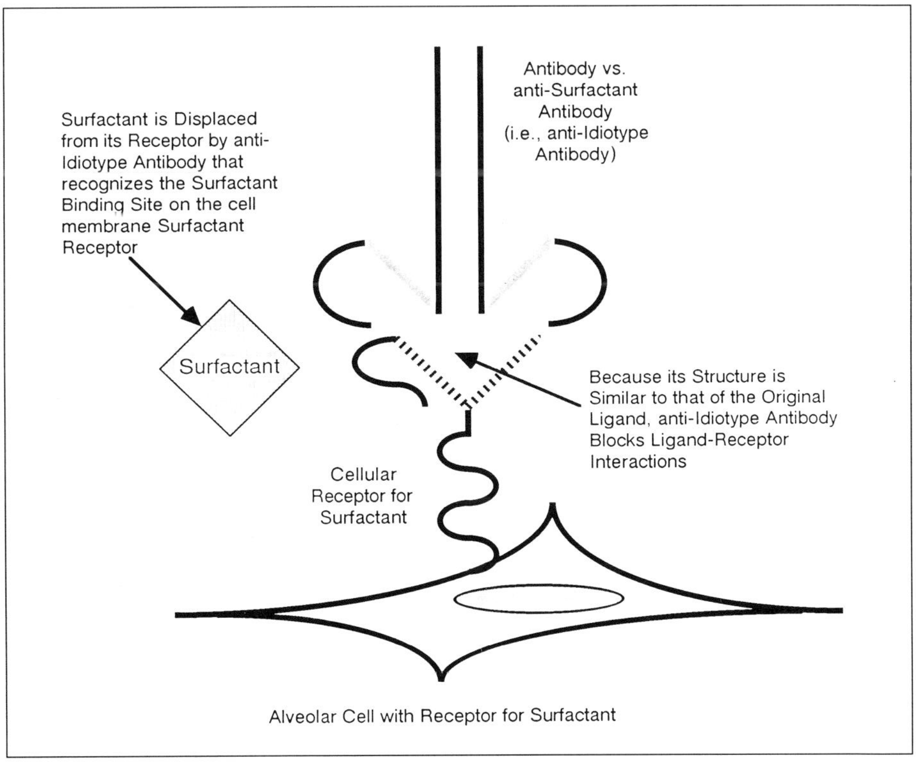
Antibody vs.
anti-Surfactant
Antibody
(i.e., anti-Idiotype
Antibody)
Surfactant is Displaced
from its Receptor by anti-
Idiotype Antibody that
recognizes the Surfactant
Binding Site on the cell
membrane Surfactant
Receptor
Surfactant
Because its Structure is
Similar to that of the Original
Ligand, anti-Idiotype Antibody
Blocks Ligand-Receptor
Interactions
Cellular
Receptor for
Surfactant
Alveolar Cell with Receptor for Surfactant

c

tor and determine its structure by sequencing this cDNA. The experiments detailed below describe our progress in this vein.

Methods

Surfactants

Curosurf was the kind gift of Drs. B. Robertson and T. Curstedt from the Karolinska Institute, Stockholm. It is composed of polar lipids, SP-B and SP-C [10]. Rabbit surfactant was prepared by ultracentrifugation of rabbit lung lavage specimens, and was the kind gift of Dr. T.A. Merritt, University of California, Davis. This preparation contains SP-A and SP-B [11]. Purified recombinant human SP-A was the kind gift of Dr. Mikko Hallman, University of California, Irvine.

Iodination

Surfactant proteins were radiolabeled with ^{125}I, using chloramine T [12]. Analysis of Curosurf iodinated in this fashion showed proteins of approximately 4, 9 and 18 kDa, and comparable analysis of rabbit surfactant showed proteins of 35, 18 and 9 kDa.

Monoclonal Antibodies to Surfactant

Fifteen monoclonal antibodies directed to Curosurf constituents and 5 monoclonal antibodies directed to rabbit surfactant were produced. These monoclonal antibodies were produced in female F344 rats using the nonsecreting rat myeloma cell line YB2/0. The production and characterization of the monoclonal anti-Curosurf antibodies are described in recent publications [13, 14]. Most of these antibodies recognize a 9-kDa protein in Curosurf. The monoclonal anti-rabbit surfactant antibodies were raised similarly, and react both with 9 and 34 kDa protein constituents (data not shown).

Anti-Idiotypic Antibodies

Anti-(anti-surfactant) monoclonal antibodies were raised against these anti-Curosurf and anti-rabbit surfactant antibodies. Female F344 rats were immunized with mixtures of monoclonal antibodies that were capable of inactivating surfactant functionally. Those antibodies used to immunize rats reacted with 9 kDa (Curosurf and rabbit surfactant) and 34 kDa (rabbit surfactant) proteins. After about 1 year of alternate week immunizations, antibody titers were noted in rats immunized to produce anti-idiotype antibodies. These anti-idiotype-producing rats were boosted, and their spleen cells fused with YB2/0 myeloma. From these experiments, one hybridoma clone (A2C) that recognized anti-Curosurf antibodies and one that recognized anti-rabbit surfactant antibodies (A2R) were isolated [15].

Immunocytochemistry

Frozen sections of human, pig and rabbit lungs were treated with normal rabbit serum, followed by A2R, A2C or YB2/0 culture supernatants. Slides were then treated with peroxidase-conjugated rabbit anti-rat IgG [16].

Western Blotting

Lung tissue was lysed, homogenized, and electrophoresed on SDS-10% PAGE. Proteins were transferred to Immobilon (Millipore Corp., Bedford, Mass.), and treated with rabbit anti-rat IgG and then with ^{125}I-*Staphylococcus* protein A (Calbiochem, La Jolla, Calif.). Reactivity was visualized by autoradiography [17].

Binding of Surfactant

Lung lavage cells from fresh porcine or rabbit lungs were washed, and incubated on ice with anti-idiotypic or control antibodies, free surfactant (1,000-fold excess relative to the amount of labeled surfactant) or saline. After washing, they were treated with 4 ng ^{125}I-labeled Curosurf or rabbit surfactant, washed again and counted in a gamma counter.

Screening of Clones

Lung cDNA expression libraries in λgt11 (Amersham, Arlington Heights, Ill.) were prepared from mRNA from homogenates of human and porcine lungs. These libraries were screened for the ability of proteins encoded by the cDNAs cloned into λgt11 to be bound by A2C and A2R by applying a combination of A2C and A2R to filters containing protein products of cloned λgt11, followed by rabbit anti-rat IgG and then ^{125}I-*Staphylococcus* protein A, according to procedures in the package insert. Positive clones, i.e. those bound by the combination of A2C and A2R, were plaque-purified twice and rescreened twice using the same approach. One independent clone was isolated from the human cDNA library and one from the porcine cDNA library in this fashion.

Genetic Analysis of cDNA Inserts

cDNA inserts had been cloned into λgt11's Eco RI site. They were therefore recovered by digestion using Eco RI, chromatography on low melting point agarose (Biorad, Richmond, Calif.) and precipitation. cDNA was radiolabeled with ^{32}P by random priming (Amers-

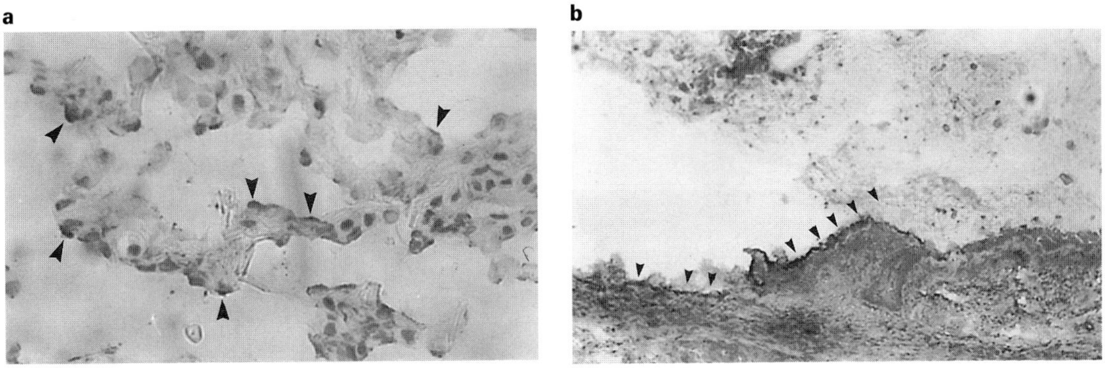

Fig. 2. Recognition of pulmonary alveolar and bronchial lining cells by anti-(anti-surfactant) antibody. **a** Binding of anti-idiotype antibody to alveolar lining cells (arrows). **b** Binding of anti-idiotype antibody to bronchial lining cells (arrows). In both cases, the rat anti-idiotype A2R is used to treat frozen sections of rabbit lung tissue. This treatment is followed by HRP-conjugated rabbit anti-rat-IgG, then diaminobenzidine as the substrate. × 1,200. From Strayer [21], with permission.

ham). Southern transfer and hybridization of these inserts was performed according to standard techniques [18]. All hybridizations were performed under conditions of relatively high stringency (50% formamide, 50 °C), and wash conditions were, similarly, of high stringency (0.2 × SSC, 42 °C).

Identification of Surfactant-Binding Activity of Proteins Produced by cDNA Clones

Phage plaques from recombinant λgt11 containing these inserts were hybridized with ^{125}I-labeled Curosurf or rabbit surfactant proteins according to established protocols [7]. Binding to surfactant was visualized by autoradiography.

Binding of Surfactant Protein to Recombinant Surfactant-Binding Protein

Escherichia coli, strain Y1090, was infected with recombinant λgt11 containing cDNA encoding the human surfactant-binding protein. Lysogenic phage colonies were isolated as described [19]. Selected lysogenic phage colonies in Y1090 were grown in broth and their production of the protein induced by IPTG [20]. Crude protein preparations from lysates of these bacteria were made [19]. electrophoresed in SDS-10% PAGE, transferred to Immobilon and hybridized with ^{125}I-SP-A.

Results

Anti-Idiotype Antibodies

Monoclonal antibody A2C recognized a series of monoclonal anti-Curosurf antibodies. Monoclonal antibody A2R recognized a series of monoclonal antibodies directed to rabbit surfactant. These two monoclonal anti-idiotype antibodies both inhibited the abilities of anti-surfactant antibodies to bind radiolabeled surfactants (data not shown). Therefore, it was concluded that A2C and A2R recognize the idiotypic, or antigen-binding, regions of anti-Curosurf and anti-rabbit surfactant antibodies.

Recognition of Pulmonary Cells by A2C and A2R

The ability of these anti-idiotype antibodies to bind lung cells was then examined. Sections of porcine and rabbit lungs were exposed to A2C and A2R, respectively, followed by horseradish-peroxidase (HRP)-conjugated rabbit anti-rat IgG. Both A2C and A2R recognize alveolar lining cells when used in this fashion (fig. 2). They do not recognize

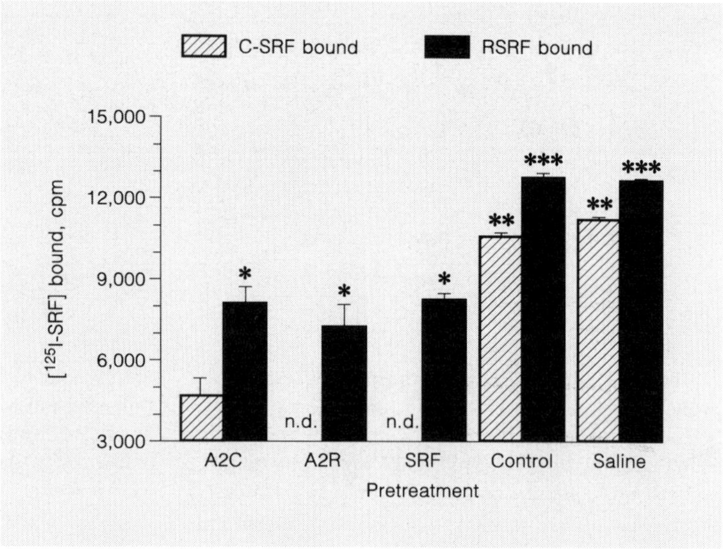

Fig. 3. Effect of pretreatment of lung lavage cells with A2C or A2R on the ability of these cells to bind ^{125}I-labeled surfactant (^{125}I-SRF). Normal pulmonary alveolar lavage cells from pigs or rabbits were pretreated with A2C, A2R, unlabeled homologous surfactant, normal saline or nothing. After pretreatment, the ability of these cells to bind ^{125}I-labeled homologous surfactant was measured. The cpm labeled surfactant bound are shown; Curosurf (C-SRF) binding to porcine lung cells by bars with diagonal hatching and rabbit SRF (RSRF) binding to rabbit lung cells by dark bars, ± SEM. n.d. = Not done. * No statistically significant difference ($p > 0.05$) between these groups; ** statistically significant difference ($p = 0.01$) between these groups and those designated by *; *** statistically significant difference ($p << 0.01$) between these groups and the A2C-pretreated porcine lung cells.

lymphocytes or macrophages, fibroblasts or endothelial cells. However, both antibodies bind to the surface of bronchial lining cells. This binding is specific, and is inhibited by preincubation of the slides with homologous surfactant [21]. Therefore, monoclonal antibodies raised against monoclonal antibodies to surfactant recognize a cell membrane structure on pulmonary alveolar lining cells and this binding is inhibited by excess free surfactant.

Inhibition of Surfactant to Pulmonary Lavage Cells

The ability of surfactant to bind specifically to pulmonary cells provides a measure of the affinity of surfactant for the surfactant receptor. The ability of A2C and/or A2R to inhibit this interaction would reflect the degree to which these anti-idiotype antibodies bind a surfactant-binding site on these pulmonary cells. Alveolar lavage cells from porcine or rabbit lungs were prepared by vigorous lavage and included bronchial and alveolar lining cells, macrophages and lymphoid cells

[21]. Preparations of pulmonary lavage cells were preincubated with A2R, A2C, 1,000-fold excess unlabeled homologous surfactant, or normal saline. They were then exposed to ^{125}I-labeled homologous surfactant, and the ability of these preparations to alter the binding of labeled surfactant to lung cells was measured. Both A2C and A2R inhibit this binding, and do so comparably to unlabeled surfactant (fig. 3).

Protein Species Bound by A2C and A2R

To identify protein species recognized by these two monoclonal anti-idiotype antibodies, lysates were prepared from lungs of pigs and rabbits. Proteins were electrophoresed on SDS-10% PAGE, transferred to Immobilon and the Immobilon filters exposed to A2C and A2R, respectively. Both A2C and A2R were found to bind proteins of similar size in their respective lung protein preparations: a main protein of 30 kDa and two minor proteins of 52 and 60 kDa (fig. 4). A2C also binds proteins of similar size in rabbit and human lung preparations and A2R binds proteins of comparable size in porcine and human lung lysates (data not shown).

Identification of Clones in cDNA Expression Library

cDNA expression libraries were prepared in λgt11 from mRNA from human and porcine lungs. These libraries were screened for their ability to produce protein that could be recognized by a combination of A2C and A2R. Only one unique clone was identified in each library that was recognized by the combined anti-idiotype antibodies. The human cDNA clone corresponds to an insert of 4.4 kb and the porcine clone to an insert of 1.8 kb (fig. 5). The cDNAs from these two clones partially cross-hybridize under stringent conditions (data not shown) and therefore their cDNA structures are similar.

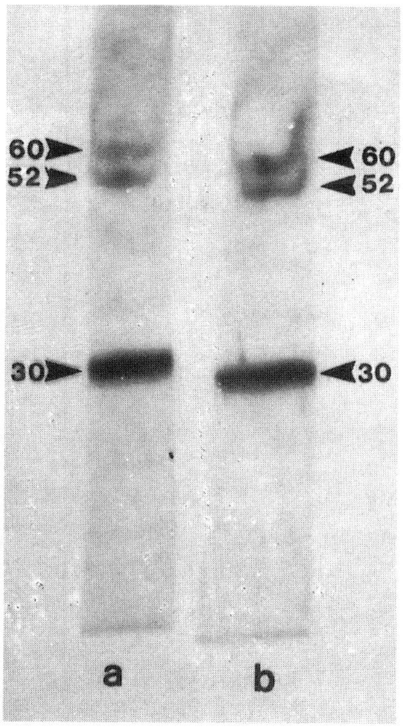

Fig. 4. Western blot profile of proteins from pulmonary cells, exposed to A2C or A2R. Crude cell lysates from lung lavage cells were prepared as described in 'Methods', electrophoresed in SDS-10% PAGE and transferred to Immobilon. Preparations from porcine lungs (**a**) were treated with A2C and those from rabbit lungs were treated with A2R (**b**). Thereafter, the filters were treated with ^{125}I-labeled *Staphylococcus* protein A and visualized by autoradiography. Molecular weights were determined by interpolation from co-electrophoresed molecular weight standards. From Strayer [21], with permission.

Surfactant Binding of Proteins Encoded by cDNA Clones

Plaque hybridization assays were then performed using either ^{125}I-SP-A or ^{125}I-Curosurf. Phage colonies containing the human and porcine cDNAs encoding proteins recognized by A2C and A2R were grown on *E. coli* and protein production induced by IPTG. Proteins were transferred to Immobilon and hybridized with both of the surfactant preparations: purified recombinant human SP-A or Curosurf. The proteins encoded by the hu-

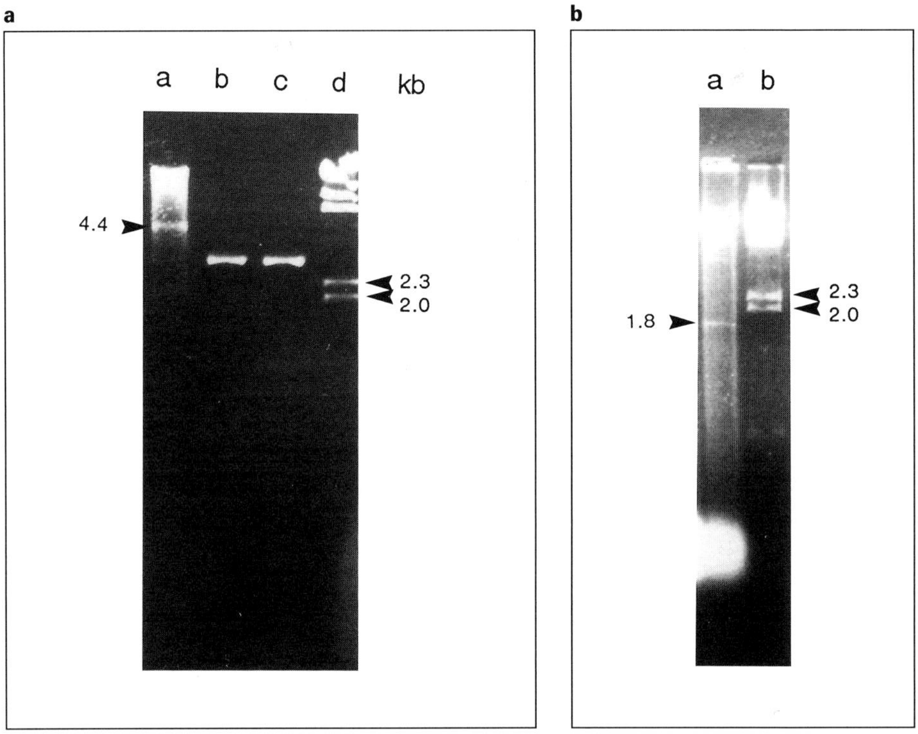

Fig. 5. cDNAs encoding SRF binding proteins in human (**a**) and porcine (**b**) cDNA expression libraries in λgt11. After screening cDNA expression libraries cloned into in λgt11 using a combination of A2C and A2R, unique clones expressing proteins recognized by these antibodies were identified and clonally purified. **a** The human cDNA insert that encodes the protein bound by these anti-idiotype antibodies corresponds to a molecular size of approximately 4.4 kb. Lane a = 4.4 kb insert; lanes b, c = pGEM7, 2.8 kb; lane d = molecular weight markers (Hind III digested λgt11). **b** The porcine insert corresponds to a molecular size of approximately 1.8 kb. Lane a = 1.8 kb insert from the porcine cDNA clone; lane b = molecular weight markers (Hind III digested λgt11).

man and porcine cDNAs both bind purified recombinant human SP-A (fig. 6). Oddly, the protein encoded by the human cDNA also bound ^{125}I-Curosurf while that encoded by the porcine cDNA did not. Neither protein bound an unrelated protein such as ovalbumin (data not shown). Therefore, the cDNA clones identified both encode proteins that bind surfactant protein A.

These cDNAs have been cloned into sequencing vectors (pGEM7), and have been partially sequenced.

The λgt11 phage containing the human cDNA encoding the SP-A binding protein was used to create lysogenic phage in *E. coli* strain Y1090. Protein preparations from these lysogeny were electrophoresed in SDS-10% PAGE, blotted to Immobilon and probed with ^{125}I-labeled purified recombinant human SP-A. Very preliminary data (fig. 7) suggest that this preparation contains a 30-kDa protein that binds SP-A.

6a 6b 6c 6d

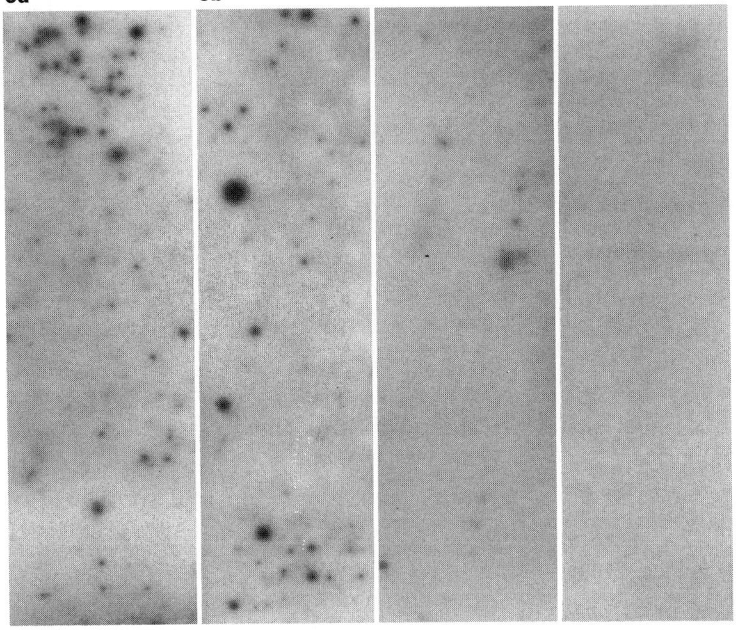

Fig. 6. Recognition of surfactant proteins by proteins encoded by cDNA from human and porcine lungs cloned into λgt11. Cloned cDNA inserts from human (**a**, **b**) or porcine (**c**, **d**) lung in λgt11 whose proteins are recognized by A2C and A2R were plated on *E. coli,* and expression induced by IPTG-impregnated Immobilon filters. These filters were then expressed to ^{125}I-labeled recombinant human surfactant protein A (**a**, **c**) or Curosurf (**b**, **d**). The protein encoded by the human clone recognizes both purified recombinant SP-A and Curosurf. That encoded by the porcine clone recognizes only SP-A.

7

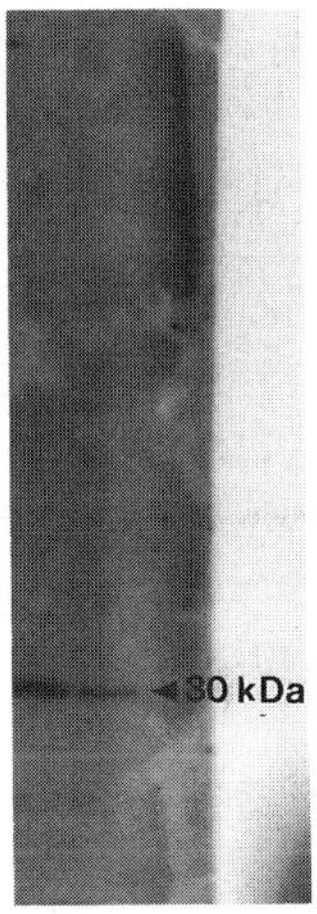

Fig. 7. Binding of SP-A by recombinant human surfactant binding protein. Protein preparations from *E. coli,* strain Y1090 made lysogenic for recombinant λgt11 containing the human surfactant binding protein cDNA, were electrophoresed, transferred to Immobilon and exposed to ^{125}I-labeled recombinant human SP-A. Molecular size was inferred from markers coelectrophoresed in parallel lanes. In this preliminary experiment, a protein of approximately 30 kDa was observed that binds SP-A. No SP-A binding is observed in the other proteins present in the bacterial lysate.

Discussion

The SP-A receptor appears to play a critical role in surfactant production and regulation. Its structural characteristics have proven elusive. The issue of identifying a surfactant receptor was therefore approached by applying the principle of molecular mimicry: two molecules that bind the same ligand are likely to have structurally related ligand-binding sites. This principle has been applied successfully to identification of receptor proteins by a number of investigators studying many different systems [22–24].

Two different anti-idiotype antibodies raised against two different anti-surfactant antibodies both recognize a 30-kDa molecule on alveolar and bronchial lining cells. These antibodies block binding of surfactant to these cells. Surfactant blocks binding of these cells by these antibodies. Thus, the 30-kDa protein is a surfactant binding protein and the two monoclonal antibodies A2C and A2R that recognize this protein bind at or near the surfactant-binding region of this protein.

The structure of this protein is not yet known. However, the combination of A2C and A2R was used to identify cDNA clones in porcine and human lung cDNA expression libraries in λgt11. The proteins produced by these libraries bind purified *recombinant* human SP-A. Finally, these two cDNAs, one from human lung and one from porcine lung, cross-hybridize to some degree but not completely. They may therefore represent different but related SP-A-binding proteins or, alternatively, unique SP-A-binding proteins with large structural differences because of their origins in different animal species. Very preliminary data suggest that the human cDNA clone encodes a 30-kDa SP-A binding protein. These experiments are being repeated making comparable protein preparations using the cloned porcine cDNA to determine the binding specificities of the proteins. In addition, the human clone is being sequenced to elucidate the structure of the encoded protein.

The function of the SP-A-binding proteins identified by these monoclonal antibodies is unknown. The effects of the 30-kDa protein on surfactant production or metabolism and its role (if any) in surfactant-related cellular activation have not been examined. However, the 30-kDa cell membrane protein [21] binds alveolar surfactant, specifically SP-A, and is present in cells known to produce and bind this protein. In this sense, it may be considered to be an SP-A receptor. The possibility that this protein may be complexed with other proteins to form a transmembrane receptor complex is under study. Such a possibility is suggested by the presence of minor bands in the Western blot preparations at 52 and 60 kDa. These could represent, e.g., a homodimer and a partial proteolytic degradation product thereof.

The present data suggest that both alveolar cells and bronchial lining cells possess this SP-A-binding protein. Though the latter have not been previously reported to participate in surfactant recycling, these cells have extensive surface elaborations providing a large surface area. This kind of arrangment would facilitate surfactant binding and prevent loss of surfactant from the lung. Studies using radiolabeled dipalmitoylphosphatidylcholine report that $<5\%$ of all surfactant escapes the lungs into the digestive tract [25]. This degree of surfactant trapping within the lung requires a very efficient surfactant binding system, and the presence of the 30 kDa protein on bronchial as well as alveolar lining cells could reasonably be consistent with this observation.

The mechanisms by which surfactant secretion is regulated appear to be quite complex. They also depend upon the operational definition of 'surfactant' used by individual investigators: for some it is surfactant protein transcription or production, while for others it is phospholipid production. The importance of SP-A binding to its receptor in the regulation of surfactant production is well documented [26]. An increasing number of other factors also appear to be important, physiologically and/or ontogenetically, in determining how much alveolar surfactant is produced.

Glucocorticoids increase phospholipid production [27] and transcription of SP-B and SP-C [28] during ontogeny. Their effects on SP-A transcription during fetal development are much more complex [29]. In cultured type II cell carcinoma lines, glucocorticoids increase transcription of SP-B [30].

Surfactant production has been reported to be regulated by receptor-mediated recognition of substances other than surfactant as well. Vasopressin stimulates phosphatidylcholine secretion in cultured rat type II pneumocytes. This stimulation reflects receptor activation [31]. Purinergic receptors also appear to regulate surfactant secretion. Adenosine A_1 and A_2 receptors on type II cells have been reported respectively to inhibit and promote phosphatidylcholine synthesis [32, 33]. The means by which purinergic receptor-mediated regulation occurs have been studied. Roles for intracellular calcium mobilization, phosphatidylinositol hydrolysis and protein kinase C activation have been described in these processes [34–36].

Therefore, regulation of surfactant production appears to be complicated. There may be differences between the predominant regulatory mechanisms as expressed during ontogeny, normal physiologic homeostasis and various pathophysiologic states. Transcription of individual surfactant proteins need not be regulated in tandem. Protein transcription and translation and phospholipid secretion may be different indices of surfactant production and may not necessarily respond in a coordinated fashion or to the same stimuli.

It is possible that identification of an SP-A-binding protein and its cDNA on alveolar lining cells will provide the means to understand an important mechanism that controls surfactant secretion. Manipulation of this regulatory apparatus could be lead to the ability to treat disorders of surfactant deficiency or excess.

Acknowledgments

This work depended greatly on the technical support of Chun-Chee Lee, Dr. Xuan Cai and Chido Makunike. Drs. Bengt Robertson and Tore Curstedt kindly provided us with Curosurf, Dr. T. Allen Merritt with rabbit surfactant and Dr. Mikko Hallman with recombinant human SP-A. Dr. Su-Ming Hsu assisted us with the immunohistochemical preparations. Thoughtful discussions with and comments from Drs. M. Hallman, A. Jobe, T.A. Merritt, B. Robertson, R. Spragg and J.R. Wright are greatly appreciated. In addition, the author thanks Dr. Jon Morrow, Associate Editor of *The American Journal of Pathology* for permission to reprint some illustrations previously published there. This work was supported by grants FD-R-000112 and FD-R-000461 from the USFDA.

References

1 Wright JR, Clements JA: Metabolism and turnover of lung surfactant. Am Rev Respir Dis 1987;135:426–444.

2 Revak SD, Merritt TA, Degryse E, Stefani L, Courtney M, Hallman M, Cochrane CG: Use of human surfactant low molecular weight apoproteins in the reconstitution of surfactant biologic activity. J Clin Invest 1988;81:826–833.

3 Yu SH, Chung W, Olafson RW, Harding PGR, Possmayer F: Characterization of the small hydrophobic proteins associated with pulmonary surfactant. Biochim Biophys Acta 1987;921:437–448.

4 Crouch E, Rust K, Persson A, Mariencheck W, Moxley M, Longmore W: Primary translation products of pulmonary surfactant protein D. Am J Physiol 1991;260:L247–L253.

5 Hawgood S, Benson BJ, Hamilton RL: Effects of a surfactant-associated protein and calcium ions on the structure and surface activity of lung surfactant lipids. Biochemistry 1985;24:184–190.

6 Notter RH, Shapiro DL, Ohning B, Whitsett JA: Biophysical activity of synthetic phospholipids combined with purified lung surfactant 6,000 dalton apoprotein. Chem Phys Lipids 1987;44:1–17.

7 Kuroki K, Mason RJ, Voelker DR: Alveolar type II cells express a high-affinity receptor for pulmonary surfactant protein A. Proc Natl Acad Sci USA 1988;85:5566–5570.

8 Wright JR, Borchelt JD, Hawgood S: Lung surfactant apoprotein SP-A (26-36 kDa) binds with high affinity to isolated alveolar type II cells. Proc Natl Acad Sci USA 1989;86:5410-5414.

9 Ryan RM, Morriss RE, Rice WR, Ciraolo G, Whitsett JA: Binding and uptake of pulmonary surfactant protein (SP-A) by pulmonary type II epithelial cells. J Histochem Cytochem 1989;37:429–440.

10 Curstedt T, Jörnwall H, Robertson B, Bergman T, Berggren P: Two hydrophobic low-molecular-mass protein fractions of pulmonary surfactant. Eur J Biochem 1987;168:255–262.
11 Hallman M, Merritt TA, Schneider H: Isolation of human surfactant from amniotic fluid and a pilot study of its efficacy in respiratory distress syndrome. Pediatrics 1983; 71:473–482.
12 Talmadge DW, Claman HN: External labeling of proteins with I^{131}, I^{125}, and I^{130}; in Williams CA, Chase MW (eds): Methods in Immunology and Immunochemistry. New York, Academic Press, 1967, pp 389–391.
13 Strayer DS, Hallman M, Merritt TA: Immunogenicity of surfactant. I. Human alveolar surfactant. Clin Exp Immunol 1991;83:35–40.
14 Strayer DS, Hallman M, Merritt TA: Immunogenicity of surfactant. II. Porcine and bovine surfactants. Clin Exp Immunol 1991;83:41–46.
15 Strayer DS, Merritt TA, Makunike C, Hallman M: Antigenicity of low molecular weight surfactant protein. Am J Pathol 1989;134:723–732.
16 Hsu SM, Raine L, Fanger H: Use of avidin-biotin-peroxidase complex (ABC) in immunoperoxidase techniques: A comparison between ABC and unlabeled antibody (PAP) procedures. J Histochem Cytochem 1981;29:577–580.
17 Towbin H, Staheiln T, Gordon J: Electrophoretic transfer of proteins from polyacrylamide gels to nitrocellulose sheets: Procedure and some applications. Proc Natl Acad Sci USA 1979;76:4350–4354.
18 Maniatis T, Fritsch EF, Sambrook J: Molecular Cloning: A Laboratory Manual. Cold Spring Harbor, Cold Spring Harbor Laboratory, 1982.
19 Singh H: Detection, purification and characterization of cDNA clones encoding DNA-binding proteins; in Ausubel FM, et al (eds): Current Protocols in Molecular Biology. New York, Wiley, 1991, pp 12.7.1–12.7.10.
20 Huynh T, Young R, Davis R: Constructing and screening cDNA libraries in λgt10 and λgt11; in Glover D (ed): DNA Cloning: A Practical Approach. Oxford, IRL Press, 1984.
21 Strayer DS: Identification of a cell membrane protein that binds alveolar surfactant. Am J Pathol 1991; 138:1085–1095.
22 Greene MI, Co MS: Shared structural features of an internal image bearing monoclonal anti-idiotype and the external antigen. Monogr Allergy 1987;22:120–125.
23 Greene MI, Kokai Y, Gaulton GN, Powell MB, Geller H, Cohen JA: Receptor systems in tissues of the nervous system. Immunol Rev 1987;100:153–184.
24 Strayer DS, Vitetta ES, Kohler H: Anti-receptor antibody. I. Isolation and characterization of the immunoglobulin receptor for phosphorylcholine. J Immunol 1975;114:722–727.
25 Pettenazzo A, Jobe A, Humme J, Seidner S, Ikegami M: Clearance of surfactant phosphatidylcholine via the upper airways in rabbits. J Appl Physiol 1988;65:2151–2155.
26 Kuroki Y, Mason RJ, Voelker DR: Chemical modification of surfactant protein A alters high affinity binding to rat alveolar type II cells and regulation of phospholipid secretion. J Biol Chem 1988;263:17596–17602.
27 Guettari N, Marin L, Bourbon J, Dufour ME, Rieutort M, Tordet C: Effects of the antiglucocorticoid RU 486 on the maturation of fetal rat lung surfactant. Exp Lung Res 1989;15:151–166.
28 Liley HG, White RT, Warr RG, Benson BJ, Hawgood S, Ballard PL: Regulation of messenger RNAs for the hydrophobic surfactant proteins in human lung. J Clin Invest 1989; 83:1191–1197.
29 Liley HG, White RT, Benson BJ, Ballard PL: Glucocorticoids both stimulate and inhibit production of pulmonary surfactant protein A in fetal human lung. Proc Natl Acad Sci USA 1988;85:9096–9100.
30 O'Reilly MA, Clark JC, Whitsett JA: Glucocorticoid enhances pulmonary surfactant protein B gene transcription. Am J Physiol 1991;260: L37–L43.
31 Brown LAS, Wood LH: Stimulation of surfactant secretion by vasopressin in primary cultures of adult rat type II pneumocytes. Biochim Biophys Acta 1989;1001:76–81.
32 Gobran LI, Rooney SA: Adenosine A_1 receptor-mediated inhibition of surfactant secretion in rat type II pneumocytes. Am J Physiol 1990;258:L45–L51.
33 Griese M, Bobran LI, Douglas JS, Rooney SA: Adenosine A_2-receptor-mediated phosphatidylcholine secretion in type II pneumocytes. Am J Physiol 1991;260:L52–L60.
34 Dorn CC, Rice WR, Singleton FM: Calcium mobilization and response recovery following P_2-purinoreceptor stimulation of rat isolated alveolar type II cells. Br J Pharmacol 1989;97:163–170.
35 Rice WR, Dorn CC, Singleton FM: P_2-purinoreceptor regulation of surfactant phophatidylcholine secretion. Biochem J 1990;266:407–413.
36 Warburton D, Buckley S, Cosico L: P1 and P2 purinergic receptor signal transduction in rat type II pneumocytes. J Appl Physiol 1989;66:901–905.

Original Paper

Biol Neonate 1992;61(suppl 1):15–20

Per Berggren[a]
Jonas Eklind[b]
Bim Linderholm[a]
Bengt Robertson[a]

[a] Research Unit for Experimental Perinatal Pathology, St. Göran's Hospital,
[b] Carl Zeiss AB, Stockholm, Sweden

Bubbles and Computer-Aided Image Analysis for Evaluation of Surfactant Inhibition

Key Words
Pulmonary surfactants
Proteins
Image analysis

Abstract
Surfactant (Curosurf, diluted to 5 mg/ml) was suspended in normal saline with 3 m*M* $CaCl_2$ and mixed with different concentrations of albumin or fibrinogen. The samples were vortexed to generate microbubbles, and the equivalent circle diameter of these bubbles was determined with computer-aided image analysis. Bubbles in the original surfactant suspension had an average diameter of 27 μm after 2 min, and their size increased only little during a 15-min period of observation. The diameter of bubbles generated in the presence of albumin (4 or 40 mg/ml) or fibrinogen (4 mg/ml) was 4–5 times larger, indicating surfactant inhibition. We conclude that evaluation of microbubble stability with image analysis provides an objective and rapid assessment of surfactant inhibition, and we speculate that the method could also be used for quantification of surfactant activity in airway samples.

Introduction

Pattle [1] discovered that fluid squeezed from the cut surface of adult lungs contains stable microbubbles and postulated the existence of a surface-tension-lowering agent at the air-liquid interfaces of lung alveoli. We now know that this postulate was correct and furthermore that the capacity of alveolar surfactant to reduce surface tension to very low values during surface compression can be lost by leakage of proteinaceous edema fluid into the airspaces [2]. Several serum proteins, including albumin and fibrinogen, have been identified as potential inhibitors of surfactant function [3, 4]. The purpose of the present

Dr. Per Berggren
Research Unit for Experimental Perinatal Pathology
St. Göran's Hospital
S-112 81 Stockholm (Sweden)

0006-3126/92/
0617-0015$2.75/0

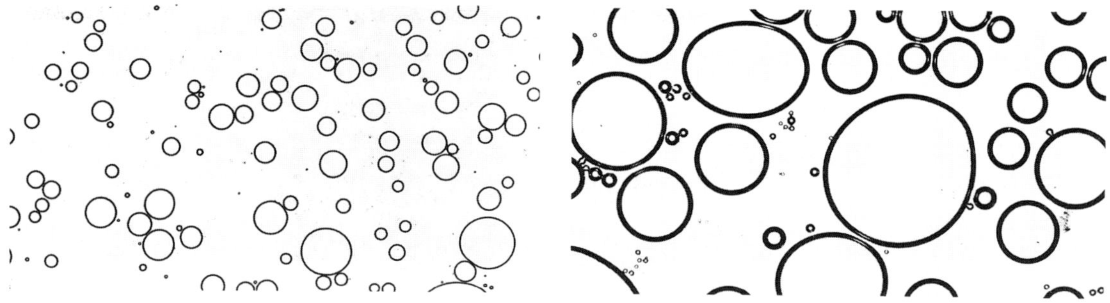

a b

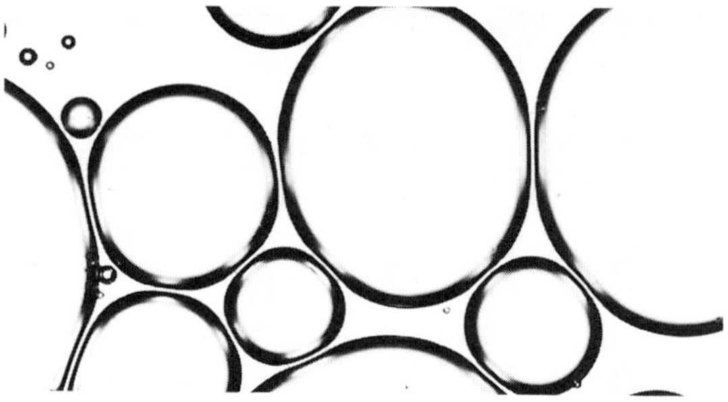

c

Fig. 1. Representative photomicrographs of bubbles in the original surfactant (**a**), and in suspensions inoculated with albumin, 40 mg/ml (**b**), or fibrinogen, 4 mg/ml (**c**). The images were obtained after 2 min. ×60.

study was to determine microbubble stability in aqueous suspensions of natural surfactant by automated image analysis, and to apply the same technique for quantification of surfactant inhibition following exposure to various concentrations of serum proteins.

Material and Methods

Surfactant (Curosurf) was prepared from minced pig lungs by washing, centrifugation, chloroform-methanol extraction and liquid gel chromatography as previously described [5]. It was suspended at a concentration of 5 mg/ml in normal saline with 3 m*M* $CaCl_2$. To the suspension we added albumin at concentrations of 4 and 40 mg/ml, or fibrinogen at concentrations of 0.4 and 4 mg/ml. These protein concentrations were chosen since for each protein they represent approximately 10 and 100%, respectively, of the normal serum concentrations. The various mixtures were incubated at room temperature for 30 min before analysis. The samples were then vortexed mechanically under standardized conditions to generate microbubbles. One drop of the sample was put on a well-slide, and examined by light microscopy at a magnification of either ×10 or ×20, depending on the size of the bubbles. The microscope was connected to a VIDAS image analyser (Kontron, Munich, FRG) via a TV camera. A specially designed program allowed us to measure the maximum and minimum diameters, and to calculate the equivalent circle diameter of the bubbles. Bubble images for analyses were obtained every second minute, 2–10 min after vortexing of the sample, and after 15 min. Representative microphotographs of bubbles in different samples are shown in figure 1a–c.

Results

Bubbles in the original surfactant suspension had similar equivalent circle diameters after 2 min and after 15 min (mean ± SEM: 27 ± 2 and 29 ± 2 μm, respectively) (fig. 2). Bubbles in the suspension incubated with the lower concentration of albumin (4 mg/ml) were significantly larger both at 2 and 15 min, indicating surfactant inhibition (107 ± 16

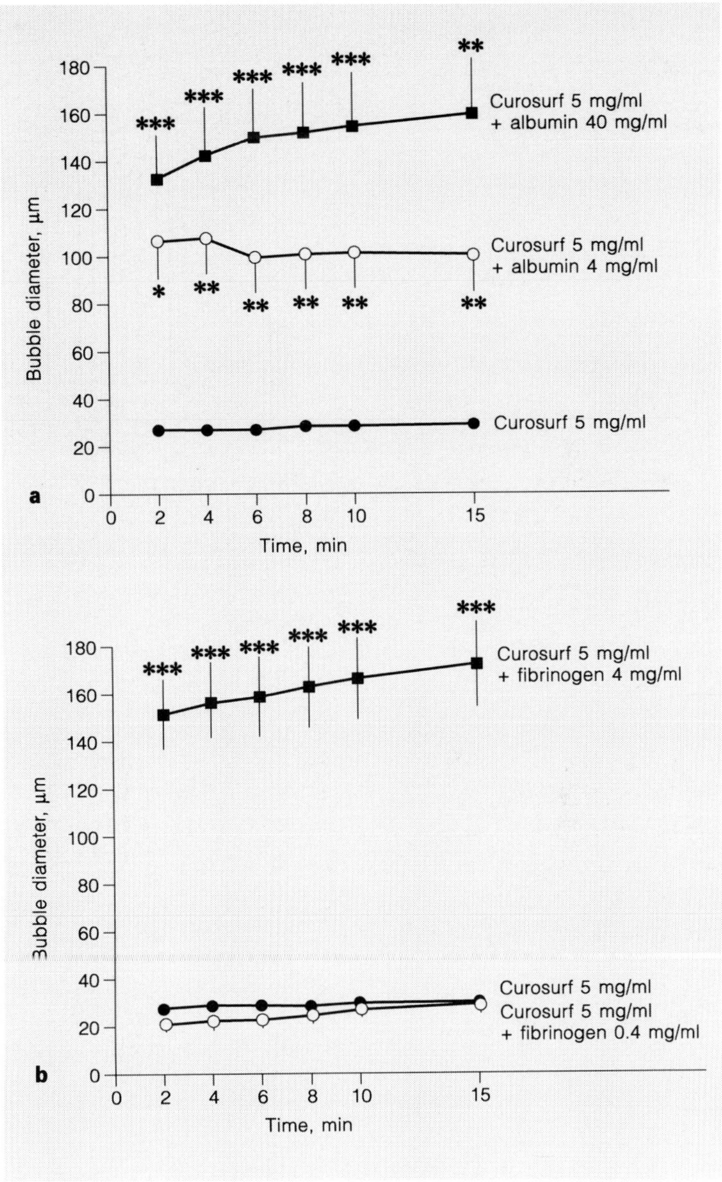

Fig. 2. Equivalent circle diameter of bubbles in the original surfactant and in suspensions inoculated with various concentrations of albumin (**a**) or fibrinogen (**b**). Values (mean, SEM) are given for various time intervals up to 15 min. *** p vs. Curosurf (**a, b**) and Curosurf + fibrinogen 0.4 mg/ml (**b**) < 0.001; ** p vs. Curosurf (**a**) < 0.01; * p vs. Curosurf (**a**) < 0.05.

and 102 ± 15 µm; p vs. original surfactant < 0.05 and 0.01, respectively). The corresponding values for bubbles in suspensions with the higher concentration of albumin (40 mg/ml) were slightly larger (133 ± 19 and 160 ± 24 µm; p vs. original surfactant < 0.001 and 0.01, respectively; p vs. lower albumin concentration NS) (fig. 2a). Bubbles in the suspension incubated with the lower concentration of fibrinogen (0.4 mg/ml) did not differ from those in original surfactant, whereas in the presence of fibrinogen at high concentra-

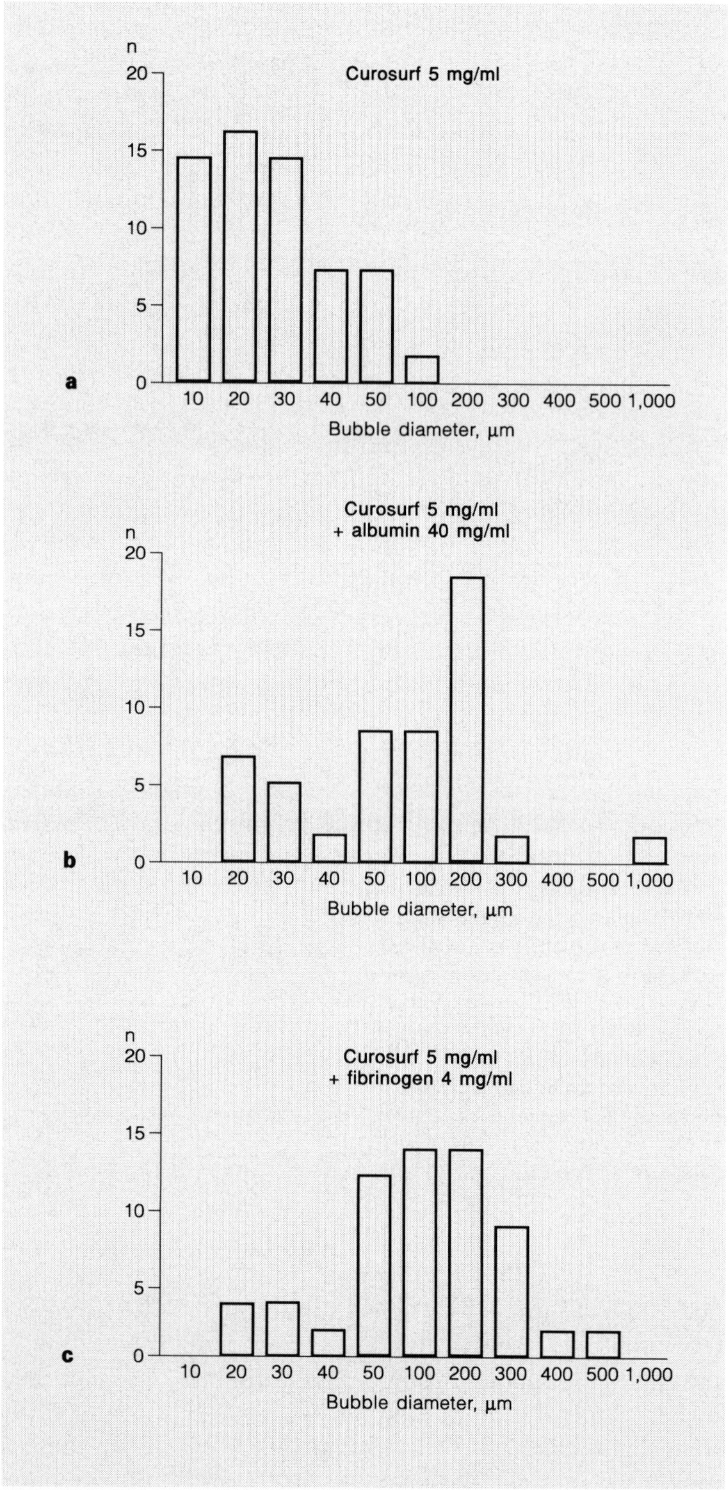

Fig. 3. Size distribution of bubbles in the original surfactant (**a**), and in suspensions inoculated with albumin, 40 mg/ml (**b**), or fibrinogen, 4 mg/ml (**c**). The values were obtained after 2 min.

tion (4 mg/ml) there was significant surfactant inhibition as indicated by markedly increased bubble diameter both at 2 and 15 min (151 ± 15 and 173 ± 19 μm; p vs. original surfactant < 0.001 at both intervals) (fig. 2b). Size distribution of bubbles in the original surfactant and in surfactant suspensions inoculated with albumin (40 mg/ml) or fibrinogen (4 mg/ml) are shown in figure 3a–c.

Discussion

Films of normal lung surfactant are characterized by very rapid adsorption to an air-liquid interface and high stability during surface compression. The first of these properties reflects the presence of specific surfactant-associated proteins (SP-A, SP-B, SP-C), and the second the high content of saturated lipids, especially dipalmitoylphosphatidylcholine, in the compressed film. Serum proteins, leaking into the alveolar spaces of an immature lung or during the course of 'adult' respiratory distress syndrome, may delay surfactant adsorption and interfere with the stability of the surface film. This, in turn, may cause alveolar instability leading to collapse or flooding of terminal airspaces with edema fluid. Inactivation of surfactant by leaking serum proteins is probably an important factor in the pathogenesis of both the neonatal [6, 7] and the adult [8] respiratory distress syndrome.

Surfactant inactivation can be evaluated under dynamic experimental conditions by in vitro methods such as the pulsating bubble [2, 3, 9, 10] or the Wilhelmy balance [4]. In the presence of surfactant inhibitors, minimum surface tension during surface compression increases, reflecting loss of film stability. Also, maximum surface tension may increase from delayed film adsorption during surface expansion. In newborn experimental animals, instillation of surfactant inhibitors into the airways causes a dose-dependent decrease in the compliance of the respiratory system, and reduced lung stability during deflation [10].

Our present data suggest that similar information on inhibitory activity can be obtained by measuring the size distribution and stability of microbubbles in samples mixed with a standard suspension of surfactant. In accordance with earlier observations [3, 4], we found that both albumin and fibrinogen have the capacity to inactivate surfactant at concentrations similar to those in serum. Albumin inactivated surfactant also at 10% of normal serum concentration, whereas this was not the case for fibrinogen. The concentration of surfactant used in the present experiments (5 mg/ml) is slightly above the 'critical concentration' of surfactant in fetal lung liquid at birth [11]. Other concentrations of surfactant in the samples might result in different sensitivity to inhibition.

We conclude that evaluation of microbubble stability with computer-aided image analysis provides an objective and rapid assessment of surfactant inhibition, and we speculate that the method, if further developed, could also be used for clinical quantification of surfactant activity in airway samples.

Acknowledgements

This work was supported by the Swedish Medical Research Council (Project 3351), Oscar II:s Jubileumsfond, and Axel Tielman's Minnesfond.

References

1 Pattle RE: Properties, function and origin of the alveolar lining layer. Nature 1955;175:1125–1126.

2 Ennema JJ, Kobayashi T, Robertson B, Curstedt T:Inactivation of exogenous surfactant in experimental respiratory failure induced by hyperoxia. Acta Anaesthesiol Scand 1988;32:665–671.

3 Fuchimukai T, Fujiwara T, Takahashi A, Enhorning G: Artificial pulmonary surfactant inhibited by proteins. J Appl Physiol 1987;62:429–437.

4 Seeger W, Stöhr G, Wolf HRD, Neuhof H: Alteration of surfactant function due to protein leakage: special interaction with fibrin monomer. J Appl Physiol 1985;58:326–338.

5 Robertson B, Curstedt T, Johansson J, Jörnvall H, Kobayashi T: Structural and functional characterization of porcine surfactant isolated by liquid-gel chromatography. Prog Respir Res 1990;25:237–246.

6 Ikegami M, Jobe A, Berry D: A protein that inhibits surfactant in respiratory distress syndrome. Biol Neonate 1986;50:121–129.

7 Jobe A: Respiratory distress syndrome – new therapeutic approaches to a complex pathophysiology. Adv Pediatr 1984;30:93–130.

8 Seeger W, Pison U, Buchhorn R, Joka T, Brand M, Obertacke U, Neuhof H, Schmit-Neuerburg K-P: Alterations in alveolar surfactant following severe multiple trauma. Prog Respir Res 1990;25:215–223.

9 Kobayashi T, Curstedt T, Grossmann G, Robertson B: Inhibition of exogenous surfactant in ventilated immature newborn rabbits. Respir Physiol 1989;76:1–12.

10 Kobayashi T, Nitta K, Ganzuka M, Inui S, Grossmann G, Robertson B: Inactivation of exogenous surfactant by pulmonary edema fluid. Pediatr Res 1991;29:353–356.

11 Kobayashi T, Shido A, Nitta K, Inui S, Ganzuka M, Robertson B: The critical concentration of surfactant in fetal lung liquid at birth. Respir Physiol 1990;80:181–192.

Original Paper

Biol Neonate 1992;61(suppl 1):21–25

Effectiveness of Curosurf for Severe Respiratory Distress Syndrome: A Case-Control Study

Adolf Valls-i-Soler
Mikel Lizarraga
Jon López de Heredia
Lourdes Roman
Edita Hernáez
Elena Gastiasoro

Neonatal Intensive Care Unit,
Perinatal Unit,
Departamento de Pediatria,
Hospital de Cruces,
Universidad del País Vasco,
Bilbao, Spain

Key Words
Pulmonary surfactants
Prematurity
Respiratory distress syndrome
Infant, newborn

Abstract
Randomized trials have proven that exogenous surfactant is effective in severe neonatal respiratory distress syndrome when strict entry criteria are applied. To evaluate efficacy of surfactant treatment in a clinical setting, we performed a case-control study. The outcome of the first 25 consecutive cases treated with porcine surfactant (Curosurf) was compared to that of 25 matched historical nontreated controls. Survival at discharge was significantly higher in surfactant-treated cases than among controls (76 vs. 48%; $p < 0.05$). No differences were found in other outcome parameters.

Introduction

Since the pioneering work of Fujiwara et al. [1], several randomized studies have demonstrated the positive effects of various exogenous surfactant preparations in the treatment of severe neonatal respiratory distress syndrome (RDS) [2–10]. In our unit, preterm infants with RDS requiring mechanical ventilation with an FiO_2 of 0.40–0.59, were randomized to be included in a clinical trial evaluating the efficacy of the early rescue treatment with porcine surfactant (Curosurf). Patients with a more severe disease ($FiO_2 \geq 0.6$) received surfactant without randomization and in order to evaluate the efficacy of surfactant treatment in these babies, a case-control study was performed. The outcome of the first consecutive 25 cases with RDS treated in our unit with surfactant outside the randomized trial was compared with that of 25 matched historical controls.

Material and Methods

Surfactant Preparation
Surfactant (Curosurf) was isolated from minced porcine lungs by a combination of washing, chloroform-methanol extraction, and liquid-gel chromatography [11]. Its composition has been described previously [12]. All batches used were supplied by Chiesi Farmaceutici (Parma, Italy).

E.G. received a research fellowship from the Department of Education of the Autonomous Bask Government.

Adolf Valls-i-Soler, MD
Unidad Neonatal
Hospital de Cruces
Universidad del País Vasco
E–48903 Barakaldo, Vizcaya (Spain)

0006–3126/92/
0617–0021$2.75/0

Patients Treated with Surfactant

Twenty-five consecutive preterm newborn infants with clinical and radiologic evidence of RDS [13], not included in the above mentioned randomized trial, were enrolled in this study from September 1989 to December 1990. The following conditions were to be met: need of mechanical ventilation, $FiO_2 \geq 0.6$, birth weight 700–2,500 g, rupture of the amniotic membranes of less that 3 days duration, no major malformations, and written informed parental consent. Patients with severe asphyxia, acidosis or a high PCO_2 were not excluded as they would have been in the randomized protocol. Intraventricular hemorrhage was not routinely ruled out before treatment. All patients were given a single dose of Curosurf (200 mg/kg, 2.5 ml/kg) by tracheal instillation. Details of the instillation procedure have been described [4].

Selection of Controls

For each of the 25 babies treated with surfactant, a historical control was chosen from a database containing the records of all RDS cases requiring mechanical ventilation in our unit from January 1987 to August 1989. None of these historical controls had received surfactant treatment. They were matched for sex, gestational age, birth weight, 1- and 5-min Apgar scores, arterial pH, and FiO_2 at admission. Controls were chosen if they were of the same sex as the corresponding case and fit all other matching criteria within a margin of 250 g for birth weight, 2 weeks for gestational age, 2 points for Apgar score, 0.2 units for arterial pH, and 0.05 for FiO_2. If more than one patient in the database fulfilled these criteria, the one closest in time to the surfactant-treated patient was selected. The medical records of surfactant-treated babies and matched controls were reviewed, and the following short term (28 days) outcomes were compared: survival at discharge from the hospital, total duration of mechanical ventilation and of supplemental oxygen administration, and incidence of the following complications: pneumothorax (PTX), pulmonary interstitial emphysema (PIE), intraventricular hemorrhage (IVH), symptomatic persistent ductus arteriosus (PDA), and bronchopulmonary dysplasia (BPD).

The diagnosis of IVH was made by ultrasound scan and graded according to criteria modified from Papile et al. [14]. The presence of a significant PDA was diagnosed from clinical and/or echocardiographic measurements [15]. BPD was defined as oxygen dependency for 28 days and/or typical radiologic findings [16].

Table 1. Characterization of patients at entry

Characteristics	Infants	
	surfactant treated (n = 25)	historical controls (n = 25)
Gestational age, weeks	29.7 ± 3.5	30 ± 2.6
Birth weight	1,375 ± 523	1,303 ± 413
1-min Apgar score	6 (1–9)	4 (1–9)
5-min Apgar score	8 (5–10)	8 (4–10)
Arterial pH	7.18 ± 0.15	7.19 ± 0.08
$PaCO_2$, mm Hg	58 ± 20	48 ± 13
FiO_2	85 ± 15	83 ± 17
A-a DO_2, mm Hg	487 ± 106	440 ± 128

Values are mean ± SD or median (range). There are no statistically significant differences between the groups.

Statistical Methods

Values are given as mean ± SD unless otherwise stated. Statistical analysis to evaluate differences between the groups was done by independent two-tailed Student's t test for continuous variables. The chi-square test was used for categorial variables. Criterion for statistical significance was a p value of 0.05 or less.

Results

Characterization of Patients

As shown in table 1, the groups were well matched for birth weight, gestational age, and 1- and 5-min Apgar scores, arterial pH, $PaCO_2$, FiO_2, and alveolar to arterial oxygen tension gradient (A-a DO_2). There were 14 male infants in each group (56%). The group of surfactant-treated babies was heterogenous in all parameters. Six of the 25 babies (24%) had a birth weight below 1,000 g, 8 (33%) and 9 (36%) had 1-min and 5-min Apgar scores less than 5 and 6, respectively. Upon admission, 9 (36%) had an arterial pH less than

Table 2. Selected outcome parameters in surfactant-treated babies and historical controls

Parameters	Surfactant-treated (n = 25)	Controls (n = 25)
Survival at discharge	19 (76%)	12 (48%)*
Pneumothorax	4 (16%)	9 (36%)
Pulmonary interstitial emphysema	5 (20%)	8 (32%)
Bronchopulmonary dysplasia	8 (32%)	6 (24%)
Intraventricular hemorrhage	11 (44%)	12 (48%)
Persistent ductus arterious	12 (48%)	16 (64%)
Mechanical ventilation, days	5 (1–26)[1]	6 (2–30)[1]
Supplemental O_2, days	14 (1–28)[1]	9 (4–31)[1]

[1] Median (range). * $p < 0.05$.

7.20, 6 (24%) a $PaCO_2$ above 60 mm Hg, and 12 (48%) had an oxygen requirement above 90 per cent. Two patients had PIE before surfactant treatment.

Comparison of Outcome

In table 2, short-term outcomes are shown for the two groups. Survival rate at discharge was significantly higher in Curosurf-treated patients than in controls (76% vs. 48%; $p < 0.05$). Differences in other outcomes did not reach statistical significance, but there are trends towards higher incidence or air leaks (PTX, PIE) in the control group, and higher incidence of BPD in surfactant-treated patients. The total time of mechanical ventilation and exposure to supplemental O_2 tended to be lower in the surfactant-treated group but these differences were not statistically significant.

Discussion

In 1981, Fuijwara et al. [1] presented the first ten cases of RDS effectively treated with surfactant. Since then, an increasing number of prospective randomized studies have demonstrated the positive effects of natural surfactant preparations of human [7, 25, 26], or heterologous [2–6, 8–10, 23, 24] origin, as well as synthetic products [17–22]. Entry criteria for these randomized trials usually excluded complicating conditions like severe perinatal asphyxia, severe PIE, and severe respiratory or metabolic acidosis. Certain factors like moderate perinatal asphyxia and very high FiO_2 requirement at entry have been associated with a poor response [27].

In contrast, in clinical practice surfactant treatment is used in many centers without strict entry criteria. Under such circumstances, babies with complicating conditions who are likely to have poor responses may be treated, and some with very severe disease will receive surfactant rather late. The outcome of these infants might differ from that in the randomized clinical trials.

In this situation, the only possible way to evaluate the effectiveness of surfactant treatment is a case-control study. We therefore compared the outcome of the first 25 consecutive nonrandomized cases treated with surfactant in our unit with that of 25 matched historical controls. Survival at discharge from the nursery was found to be higher in the surfactant-treated group whereas differences in other outcome parameters did not reach the level of statistical significance. The trend towards higher incidence of BPD in surfactant-treated babies could possibly be explained by the fact that a significantly greater number of immature babies survived in this group.

The results of more than 15 published controlled trials of surfactant replacement therapy for neonatal RDS have recently been reviewed [28, 29]. In summary, rescue trials have shown an improvement in respiratory function with a decrease in FiO_2 requirement, and a reduced incidence of pulmonary air leaks. On the whole, the mortality rate is almost halved by surfactant treatment [28]. The only side effects found in several series is an increased incidence of clinically significant PDA.

Our results appear to be similar to those in the majority of these previous trials. If we compare the outcome of the present 25 cases treated with surfactant in an uncontrolled manner with corresponding data from treated babies in the first collaborative European multicenter trial [4], we find that mortality (24 vs. 31%) and incidence figures for PIE, PTX, BPD, IHV, and PDA are indeed very similar.

We conclude that administration of a single large dose of Curosurf to a nonselected, nonrandomized population of babies with severe RDS, requiring mechanical ventilation with an $FiO_2 \geq 0.06$, significantly improved survival at discharge from our unit, in comparison with historical untreated control cases of similar severity.

References

1 Fujiwara T, Chida S, Watabe Y, Maeta H, Morita T, Abe T: Artificial surfactant treatment in hyaline membrane disease. Lancet 1980;i:55–59.

2 Raju TNK, Vidyasagar D, Bhat R, Sobel D, McCulloch KM, Anderson M, Maeta H, Levy PS, Furner S: Double-blind controlled trial of single-dose treatment with bovine surfactant in hyaline membrane disease. Lancet 1987;i:651–656.

3 Gitlin JD, Soll RF, Parad RB, Horbar JD, Feldman HA, Lucey JF, Taeusch HW: Randomized controlled trial of exogenous surfactant for the treatment of hyaline membrane disease. Pediatrics 1987;79:31–37.

4 Collaborative European Multicenter Study Group: Surfactant replacement therapy for severe neonatal respiratory distress syndrome: An international randomized clinical trial. Pediatrics 1988;82:683–691.

5 Konishi M, Fujiwara T, Naito T, Takeuchi Y, Ogawa Y, Inukai K, Fujimura M, Nakamura H, Hashimoto T: Surfactant replacement therapy in neonatal respiratory distress syndrome. A multi-centre, randomized clinical trial: Comparison of high- versus low-dose of Surfactant TA. Eur J Pediatr 1988;147:20–25.

6 Horbar JD, Soll RF, Sutherland JM, Kotagal U, Philip AGS, Kessler DL, Little GA, Edwards WH, Vidyasagar D, Raju TNK, Jobe AH, Ikegami M, Mullett MD, Myerberg DZ, McAuliffe TL, Lucey JF: A multicenter randomized, placebo-controlled trial of surfactant therapy for respiratory distress syndrome. N Engl J Med 1989;320:959–965.

7 Lang MJ, Hall RT, Reddy NS, Kurth CG, Merritt TA: A controlled clinical trial of human surfactant replacement therapy for severe respiratory distress syndrome in very low birth weight infants. J Pediatr 1990;116:295–300.

8 Soll RF, Hoekstra RE, Fangman JJ, Corbet AJ, Adams JM, James LS, Schulze K, Oh W, Roberts JD, Dorst JP, Kramer SS, Gold J, Zola EM, Horbar JD, McAuliffe TL, Lucey JF: Multicenter trial of single-dose modified bovine surfactant (Survanta) for prevention of respiratory distress syndrome. Pediatrics 1990;85:1092–1102.

9 Walti H, Relier JP, Huon C, Monset-Couchard M, Scemama M, De Gamarra E, Moriette G, Curstedt T, Robertson B: Traitement des formes sévères de la maladie des membranes hyalines par une dose unique d'un surfactant exogène naturel d'origine porcine. Un essai randomisé: Effets immédiats et devenir à 28 jours de vie. Arch Fr Pédiatr 1990;47:329–334.

10 Horbar JD, Soll RF, Schachinger M, Kewitz G, Versmold HT, Lindner W, Duc G, Mieth D, Linderkamp O, Zilow EP, Lemburg P, Von Lowenich V, Brand M, Minoli I, Moro G, Riegel KP, Roos R, Weiss L, Lucey JF: A European multicenter randomized controlled trial of single dose surfactant therapy for idiopathic respiratory distress syndrome. Eur J Pediatr 1990;149:416–423.

11 Noack G, Berggren P, Curstedt T, Grossmann G, Herin P, Mortensson W, Nilsson R, Robertson B: Severe neonatal respiratory distress syndrome treated with the isolated phospholipid fraction of natural surfactant. Acta Paediatr Scand 1987; 76:697–705.

12 Robertson B, Curstedt T, Johansson J, Jörnvall H, Kobayashi T: Structural and functional characterization of porcine surfactant isolated by liquid-gel chromatography. Prog Respir Res 1989;25:237–246.

13 Hjalmarson O: Epidemiology and classification of acute, neonatal respiratory distress: A prospective study. Acta Paediatr Scand 1981;70: 773–783.

14 Papile LA, Burstein J, Burstein R, Koffler H: Incidence and evolution of subependymal and intraventricular hemorrhage: A study of infants with birth weights less than 1500 grams. J Pediatr 1978;92:529–534.

15 Valls-Soler A, Benito J, Pastor E, López de Heredia J, Santiago M, Cabrera A: Tratamiento con Indometacina endovenosa del ductus arterioso sintomático en el recién nacido pretérmino. An Esp Pediatr 1987; 27:112–116.

16 Northway WH, Rosan RC, Porter DY: Pulmonary disease following respiratory therapy of hyaline-membrane disease. N Engl J Med 1967; 276:357–368.

17 Halliday HL, McClure G, Reid MMc, Lappin TRI, Meban C, Thomas PS: Controlled trial of artificial surfactant to prevent respiratory distress syndrome. Lancet 1984;i: 476–478.

18 Phibbs RH, Ballard RA, Clements JA, Heibron DC, Phibbs CS, Schlueter MA, Sniderman SH, Tooley WH, Wakeley A: Initial clinical trial of Exosurf, a protein-free synthetic surfactant, for the prophylaxis and early treatment of hyaline membrane disease. Pediatrics 1991;88: 1–9.

19 Ten Center Study Group: Ten center trial of artificial surfactant (artificial lung expanding compound) in very premature babies. Br Med J 1987;294:991–996.

20 Morley CJ, Greenough A, Miller NG, Bangham AD, Pool J, Wood S, South M, Davis JA, Vyas H: Randomized trial of artificial surfactant (ALEC) given at birth to babies from 23 to 34 weeks gestation. Early Hum Dev 1988;17:41–54.

21 Bose C, Corbet A, Bose G, Garcia-Prats J, Lombardy L, Wold D, Donion D, Long W: Improved outcome at 28 days of age for very low birth weight infants treated with a single dose of a synthetic surfactant. J Pediatr 1990;117:947–953.

22 Corbet A, Bucciarelli R, Goldman S, Mammel M, Wold D, Long W, the American Exosurf Pediatric Study Group. Decreased mortality rate among small premature infants treated with a single dose of synthetic surfactant: A multicenter controlled trial. J Pediatr 1991;118: 277–284.

23 Kendig JW, Notter RH, Cox C, Reubens LJ, Davis JM, Maniscalco WM, Sinkin RA, Bartoletti A, Dwerck HS, Horgan MJ, Risemberg H, Phelps DL, Shapiro DL: A comparison of surfactant as immediate prophylaxis and as rescue therapy in newborns of less than 30 weeks' gestation. N Engl J Med 1991;324:865–871.

24 Hoekstra RE, Jackson JC, Myers TF, Frantz III ID, Stern ME, Powers WF, Maurer M, Raye JR, Carrier ST, Gunkel JH, Gold AJ: Improved neonatal survival following multiple doses of bovine surfactant in very premature neonates at risk for respiratory distress syndrome. Pediatrics 1991;88:10–18.

25 Hallman M, Merritt TA, Järvenpaa AI, Boynton B, Mannino F, Gluck L, Edwards D: Exogenous human surfactant for treatment of severe RDS: A randomized prospective clinical trial. J Pediatr 1985;106: 963–969.

26 Merritt TA, Hallman M, Blood BT, Berry C, Benirschke K, Sahn D, Key T, Edwards D, Järvenpaa AL, Pohjavuori M, Kankaanpaa K, Kunnas M, Paatero H, Rapola J, Jaaskelainen J: Prophylactic treatment of very premature infants with human surfactant. N Engl J Med 1986;315: 785–790.

27 Collaborative European Multicenter Study Group: Factors influencing the clinical response to surfactant replacement therapy in babies with severe respiratory distress syndrome. Eur J Pediatr 1991; 150:433–439.

28 Morley CJ: Surfactant treatment for premature babies. A review of clinical trials. Arch Dis Child 1991;66: 445–450.

29 Committee on Fetus and Newborn, American Academy of Pediatrics: Surfactant replacement therapy for respiratory distress syndrome. Pediatrics 1991;87:946–947.

Original Paper

Biol Neonate 1992;61(suppl 1):26–30

E. Herting[a], *C.P. Speer*[a]
K. Harms[a], *B. Robertson*[b]
T. Curstedt[c], *H.L. Halliday*[d]
D. Compagnone[e], *O. Gefeller*[e]
G. McClure[d], *M. Reid*[d]
R. Tubman[d], *P. Herin*[b]
G. Noack[b], *J. Kok*[f]
J. Koppe[f], *L. van Sonderen*[f]
E. Laufkötter[g], *W. Köhler*[h]
H. Boenisch[i], *K. Albrecht*[j]
C. Roll[k], *L. Hanssler*[k]
M. Haim[l], *S.B. Oetomo*[m]
A. Okken[m], *P.C. Altfeld*[n]
P. Groneck[o], *W. Kachel*[p]
J.P. Relier[q], *H. Walti*[q]

[a] Department of Pediatrics, University of Göttingen, FRG;
[b] Research Unit for Experimental Perinatal Pathology and St. Göran's Children's Hospital, Stockholm,
[c] Department of Clinical Chemistry, Danderyd Hospital, Stockholm, Sweden;
[d] Royal Maternity Hospital, Belfast, UK;
[e] Department of Medical Statistics, University of Göttingen, FRG;
[f] Academisch Ziekenhuis, Amsterdam, The Netherlands;
[g] Departments of Pediatrics, University of Bochum,
[h] University of Bonn,
[i] Community Hospital, Braunschweig,
[j] Central Hospital, Bremen,
[k] University of Essen, FRG;
[l] University Hospital, Graz, Austria;
[m] University Hospital, Groningen, The Netherlands;
[n] Pediatric Hospital (Auf der Bult), Hannover,
[o] Pediatric Hospital Köln,
[p] Pediatric Hospital, Mannheim, FRG;
[q] University of Paris, France

Factors Influencing Morbidity and Mortality in Infants with Severe Respiratory Distress Syndrome Treated with Single or Multiple Doses of a Natural Porcine Surfactant

Key Words

Respiratory distress syndrome
Pulmonary surfactants
Infant, newborn

Abstract

In an international multicenter trial infants with clinical and radiological signs of severe RDS (age 2–15 h, birthweight 700–2,000 g, mechanical ventilation, $FiO_2 \geq 0.6$, no complicating disease) were randomized to receive either a single dose (n = 176) or up to three subsequent doses (n = 167) of a natural porcine surfactant (Curosurf). Using a logistic regression model, the effects of therapy, birthweight, sex, hospital and other clinical factors on survival and various outcome parameters were evaluated. Mortality (13 vs. 21%, $p < 0.05$) and the incidence of pneumothorax (9 vs. 18%, $p < 0.01$) were significantly lower in the multiple-dose group. Low birthweight, hospital allocation, low Apgar score and initial disease severity were associated with an increased mortality. Low birthweight, hypothermia (admission temperature <36 °C) and acidosis (pH < 7.25) prior to surfactant treatment could be identified as risk factors for the development of intracranial hemorrhage.

Egbert Herting, MD
Department of Pediatrics
University of Göttingen
Robert-Koch-Strasse 40
D-W-3400 Göttingen (FRG)

0006–3126/92/
0617–0026$2.75/0

Introduction

Surfactant replacement therapy is a major breakthrough in neonatal medicine. Various controlled studies have underlined the positive effect of natural surfactant treatment on mortality and morbidity of infants with severe RDS [1]. Apart from surfactant replacement, however, the prognosis of infants with RDS is influenced by a variety of additional factors such as birthweight, sex and standard of perinatal management [2, 3]. In this study data from a randomized multicenter trial (single versus multiple doses of surfactant) [4] were subjected to logistic regression analysis and factors influencing morbidity and mortality of infants were identified.

Methods

Surfactant. Curosurf is a natural surfactant preparation isolated from minced pig lung by a combination of washing, centrifugation, chloroform-methanol extraction and liquid gel chromatography. Curosurf contains the two low molecular weight hydrophobic apoproteins SP-B and SP-C but not SP-A [5]. The efficiency of a single dose has been shown in animal experiments [6] and in a randomized controlled trial [7].

Study Design. Fifteen European neonatal intensive care units contributed to this trial: Amsterdam, Belfast, Bochum, Bonn, Braunschweig, Bremen, Essen, Göttingen, Graz, Groningen, Hannover, Köln, Mannheim, Paris, Stockholm. Before randomization anemia, hypotension, hypoglycemia and pneumothorax were treated by appropriate measures. The entry criteria were:

(1) Birthweight 700–2,000 g.
(2) Clinical and radiological signs of severe RDS.
(3) Age at treatment 2–15 h.
(4) Requirement of mechanical ventilation.
(5) Fraction of inspiratory oxygen (FiO_2) ≥ 0.6.
(6) No severe congenital malformation.
(7) No severe asphyxia (5 min Apgar ≤ 3).

Before surfactant administration all infants were ventilated according to a standardized protocol [8]. Written informed consent was obtained from the parents. Randomization to single- or multiple-dose treatment was performed by opening sealed opaque envelopes in numerical order. Infants in the single-dose group received one dose of 200 mg/kg body weight of Curosurf. Babies randomized to multiple-dose treatment were treated with an identical initial dose but received up to two further doses of 100 mg/kg birthweight 12 and 24 h after initiation of treatment if they were still on the ventilator and needed supplemental oxygen ($FiO_2 > 0.21$).

Obstetric and perinatal data were collected using a case record form. Disease severity on chest X-ray was classified according to the criteria of Gideon et al. [9]. Pneumothorax was diagnosed clinically and radiologically. Persistent ductus arteriosus was diagnosed on clinical grounds and by echocardiography. Intracranial hemorrhages were classified on ultrasound scan according to Papile et al. [10]. Bronchopulmonary dysplasia (BPD) was assumed if the infant was still on oxygen on day 28 and had radiological changes compatible with chronic lung disease [11]. Mortality and the incidence of complications were evaluated on day 28.

The study was approved by each local hospital or university ethical committee.

Statistics. Differences between the groups were evaluated by the Wilcoxon and the χ^2 test. The level of statistical significance was defined as $p < 0.05$. To analyse the impact of factors other than multiple-dose treatment on survival and morbidity, we used a logistic regression model. Categories for continuous variables (e.g. birthweight 700–1,200 and 1,201–2,000 g) were also introduced. The relative risk between groups of developing a certain complication was expressed using the odds ratio (OR). An odds ratio < 1 describes a reduced risk, and if the upper limit of the 95% confidence interval (CI) is also < 1 statistical significance can be assumed at the 5% level [12, 13].

Results

Characterization of Patients. One hundred and seventy-six patients were randomized to receive a single dose, and 167 patients to receive multiple-dose treatment. There were no significant differences in baseline data between the groups. The patients were well matched for gestational age (mean $\pm$ SD: 29.2 $\pm$ 2.5, 28.9 $\pm$ 2.2 weeks), birthweight (1,218 $\pm$ 327, 1,189 $\pm$ 321 g), sex (56.3%, 54.5% males), age of treatment (median: 6.0, 6.7 h) and disease severity at randomization

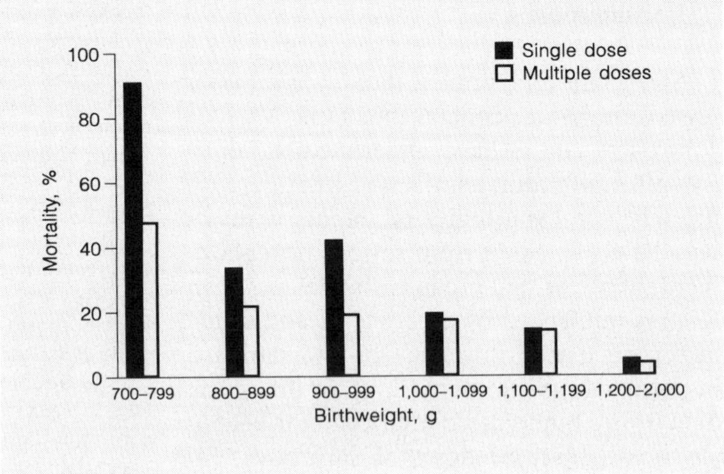

Fig. 1. 28-day mortality (%) and birthweight (g) following single- or multiple-dose treatment. Birthweight is plotted in steps of 100 g up to 1,199 g; the higher birthweight babies (1,200–2,000 g) are combined on the right of the figure.

(median FiO_2:0.83, 0.90). In the multiple-treatment group, 109/167 patients (65%) required additional surfactant doses. Oxygenation immediately improved after instillation of surfactant and there was a reduction of ventilatory requirements. From day 2 to day 4 after surfactant treatment peak inspiratory pressure, mean airway pressure and frequency were lower in the multiple-dose group compared to the single-dose group [4].

Twenty-Eight-Day Outcome and Logistic Regression Analysis. Infants in the multiple-treatment group had a lower incidence of pneumothorax (18 vs. 9%, $p < 0.001$) and a lower mortality (21 vs. 13%, $p < 0.05$). The combined incidence of mortality and BPD on day 28 was 33% in the single-dose group and 27% in the multiple-dose group ($p = 0.08$). There were no significant differences of pulmonary and extrapulmonary complications, duration of artificial ventilation or time of total exposure to oxygen between the two groups.

Logistic regression analysis confirmed the effects of therapy, birthweight and gender on 28-day outcome. Low birthweight (≤ 1,200 g) was associated with a significantly increased incidence of intracranial hemorrhage (OR: 0.33, CI: 0.20–0.55, $p < 0.001$) and BPD (OR: 0.36, CL: 0.17–0.76, $p < 0.01$) and increased mortality (OR: 0.05, CI: 0.02–0.16, $p < 0.001$). Mortality was high in the group of lightest babies (700–799 g) (fig. 1). Significantly fewer girls than boys died or developed BPD (OR: 0.49; CI: 0.27–0.90, $p < 0.05$).

Additionally, hospital allocation had a strong influence on mortality; the differences in 28-day mortality between the 8 biggest centers in the trial are depicted in figure 2.

Using the logistic regression model, we could identify the influence of disease severity on survival as judged by chest radiograph grading [9]. Significantly more infants with RDS grade I-III survived as compared to infants with RDS grade IV ($p < 0.05$). Perinatal management and condition of the infants at birth were shown to influence survival. Low Apgar-score at 5 min (≤6) was associated with a decreased survival rate (fig. 3).

Hypothermia (rectal temperature at admission < 36 °C), and acidosis before surfactant treatment (pH < 7.25) were both associated with a higher incidence of intracranial hemorrhage ($p < 0.05$).

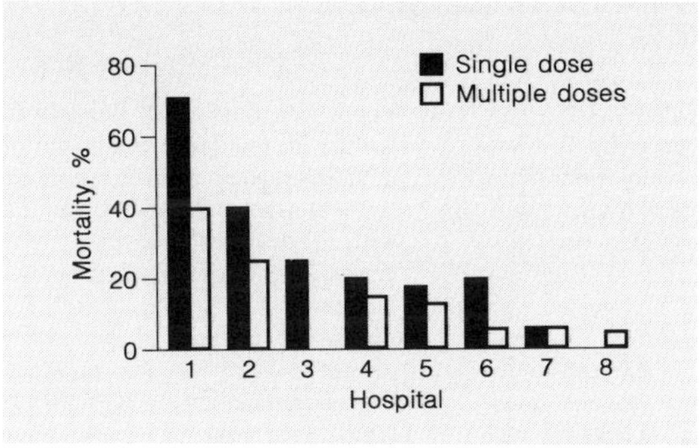

Fig. 2. 28-day mortality (%) and hospital allocation in infants treated with a single or multiple doses of surfactant. The 8 biggest hospitals in the trial were coded by numbers (1–8).

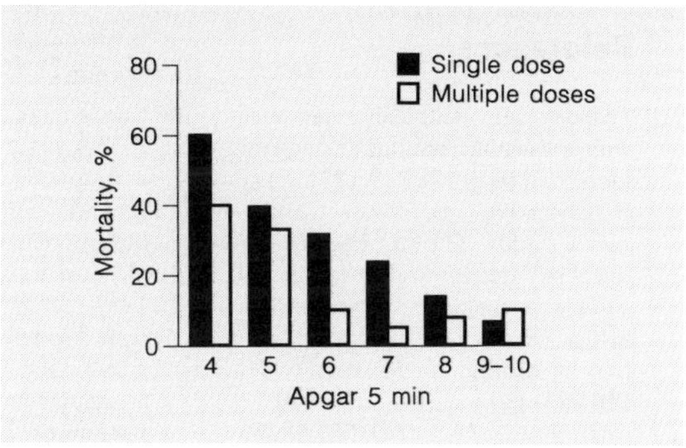

Fig. 3. 28-day mortality (%) and Apgar score at 5 min.

The following variables did not significantly influence the outcome of infants: maternal steroid treatment, inborn or outborn status, presence of a neonatologist at birth, duration of transport, hemoglobin concentration at admission, or blood pressure just prior to surfactant treatment.

Discussion

In our study, mortality and the incidence of pneumothorax in infants with severe RDS were significantly reduced by multiple-dose treatment as compared to a single-dose regimen [4]. Apart from surfactant treatment, 28-day outcome of infants with severe RDS was influenced by various clinical factors. Low birthweight turned out to be the strongest risk factor. Mortality and the incidence and severity of intracranial hemorrhage were strikingly higher in babies with a birthweight below 1,200 g. The data of our study suggest that every effort should be made to avoid perinatal asphyxia, acidosis and hypothermia. Since disease severity was shown to influence outcome of patients, surfactant substitution at an earlier stage of disease could be considered a possible advantage for further reducing mortality. The striking differences in mortality and morbidity between individual centers suggest that apart from local circumstances (socio-economic factors, admission policies, structure of the unit, etc.), there might be differences in the management of infants at risk. Clearly, the role of mechanical ventilation, fluid intake, nutritional status and other supportive measures of neonatal intensive care has to be evaluated and defined. Although the optimal therapeutic regimen for surfactant replacement in severe RDS still needs to be identified, the results of this trial underline the importance of an optimal pre- and perinatal management of infants at risk.

Acknowledgement

This work was supported by a grant from the German government (BMFT 93-607-27).

References

1 Halliday HL: Clinical experience with exogenous natural surfactant. Dev Pharmacol 1989;13:173–181.

2 Collaborative European Multicenter Study Group: Factors influencing the clinical response to surfactant replacement therapy in babies with severe respiratory distress syndrome. Eur J Pediatr 1991; 150:433–439.

3 Charon A, Taeusch HW, Fitzgibbon C, Smith GB, Treves ST, Phelps DS: Factors associated with surfactant treatment response in infants with severe respiratory distress syndrome. Pediatrics 1989;83:348–354.

4 Speer CP, Robertson B, Curstedt T, Halliday HL, Compagnone D, Gefeller G, Harms K, Herting E, McClure G, Reid M, Tubman R, Herin P, Noack G, Kok G, Koppe J, van Sonderen L, Laufkötter E, Köhler W, Boenisch H, Albrecht K, Hanssler L, Haim M, Oetomo SB, Okken A, Altfeld PC, Groneck P, Kachel W, Relier JP, Walti H: Randomized European multicenter trial of surfactant replacement therapy for severe neonatal respiratory distress syndrome: Single versus multiple doses of Curosurf. Pediatrics 1992;89:13–20.

5 Curstedt T, Jörnvall H, Robertson B, Bergmann T, Berggren P: Two hydrophobic low-molecular-mass protein fractions of pulmonary surfactant: Characterization and biophysical activity. Eur J Biochem 1987;168:255–262.

6 Robertson B, Curstedt T, Johannson J, Jörnvall H, Kobayashi T: Structural and functional characterization of procine surfactant isolated by liquid-gel chromatography. Prog Respir Res 1989;238:246.

7 Collaborative European Multicenter Study Group: Surfactant replacement therapy for severe neonatal respiratory distress syndrome: an international randomized clinical trial. Pediatrics 1989;82:683–691.

8 Speer CP, Harms K, Herting E, Neumann N, Curstedt T, Robertson B: Early and late surfactant replacement therapy in severe respiratory distress syndrome. Lung 1990; 168(suppl):870–876.

9 Giedion A, Haefliger H, Dangel P: Acute pulmonary X-ray changes in hyaline membrane disease treated with artificial ventilation and positive end-exspiratory pressure (PEEP). Pediatr Radiol 1973;1:145.

10 Papile LA, Burstein J, Burstein R, Koffler H: Incidence and evolution of subependymal and intraventricular hemorrhage: A study of infants with birthweight less than 1500 grams. J Pediatr 1978;92:529–534.

11 Northway WH Jr, Rosan RC: Radiographic features of pulmonary oxygen toxicity in the newborn: bronchopulmonary dysplasia. Radiology 1968;91:49–58.

12 Kleinbaum DG, Kupper LL, Chambless LE: Logistic regression analysis of epidemiologic data: Theory and practice. Commun Statist Theor Meth 1982;11:485–547.

13 Bartolucci AA, Fraser MD: Comparative step-up and composite tests for selecting prognostic indicators associated with survival. Biometrical J 1977;19:437–448.

Original Paper

Biol Neonate 1992;61(suppl 1):31–36

Liselotte Skov
Angela Bell
Gorm Greisen

Department of Neonatalogy,
University Hospital Rigshospitalet,
Copenhagen, Denmark

Surfactant Administration and the Cerebral Circulation

Key Words
Pulmonary surfactants
Electroencephalography
Near infrared spectroscopy
Cerebrovascular circulation
Cerebral blood volume
Cerebral blood flow

Abstract
We have used two main techniques to investigate the effect of surfactant therapy on the cerebral circulation in 34 babies. Twenty-one babies were studied using near infrared spectroscopy and 13 had cerebral blood flow measured using a xenon clearance technique. Other measures recorded included amplitude integrated EEG, mean arterial blood pressure and central venous or oesophageal pressure. There was a marked depression in EEG activity lasting for 10–20 min after surfactant administration. Cerebral blood volume and cerebral blood flow were maintained in most infants in spite of a fall in mean arterial blood pressure. We conclude that factors other than cerebral ischaemia cause the transient disturbance in electrophysiologic activity.

Introduction

Treatment of premature infants with porcine surfactant (Curosurf) for severe respiratory distress syndrome (RDS) results in a marked reduction in mortality and morbidity [1]. RDS and intraventricular haemorrhage (IVH) are common complications of prematurity which are stronlgy associated, but despite this, no consistent reduction in the risk of IVH has been documented following surfactant therapy [2]. Studies of the acute effects of surfactant therapy on the cerebral circulatory system have given conflicting results [3–11].

We have previously noted a depression of EEG activity following administration of natural surfactant (Curosurf), concurrent with a fall in mean arterial blood pressure (MABP) [4]. We therefore planned to study the cerebral circulatory system using two different techniques: near infrared spectroscopy (NIRS) for monitoring changes in cerebral blood volume (CBV) and ^{133}Xe-clearance for measuring changes in cerebral blood flow (CBF) to look for evidence of acute cerebral

Dr. Liselotte Skov
Department of Neonatology (GN 5024)
Rigshospitalet
Blegdamsvej 9
DK–2100 Copenhagen (Denmark)

0006–3126/92/
0617–0031$2.75/0

ischaemia as the cause of the EEG depression. Some of the data summarized here have been described in detail elsewhere [3, 4].

Material and Methods

Patients

The criteria for surfactant treatment were as in the European multicenter study [1], except that babies were enrolled up to 48 h postnatal age. Thirty-four babies admitted to the Department of Neonatalogy at Rigshospitalet in Copenhagen were studied during treatment with natural surfactant. Twenty-one babies were studied using NIRS and, in an ongoing study, 13 other babies had CBF measured using a xenon clearance technique. MABP was measured in all babies. Central venous pressure (CVP) or oesophageal pressure (OP) was measured in 10 babies (CVP in 2 and OP in 8). Twenty-eight babies had continuous amplitude-integrated EEG (aEEG) monitoring. The babies had a mean birth weight of 1,305 g (range 645–2,560 g) and a mean gestational age of 29 weeks (range 25–34 weeks). Median age at treatment was 12.5 h (range 4–48 h).

Administration of Surfactant

A bolus of 200 mg/kg body weight of porcine surfactant suspended in saline (Curosurf, 80 mg/ml) was instilled into the endotracheal tube via a feeding catheter placed with the tip just above the carina. Some babies received the surfactant by half-dose instillation in each lung, and others received the surfactant in one bolus dose lying supine. Manual ventilation after instillation was not performed. The babies were reconnected to the ventilator and the ventilator settings were modified according to the clinical response.

Oesophageal Pressure and Central Venous Pressure

OP was measured by a feeding tube lying in the oesophagus connected to a transducer and CVP was measured from an umbilical venous catheter. Although these pressures are not directly comparable, they should both be sensitive to a significant increase in intrathoracic pressure, resulting from a sudden increase in lung compliance and/or functional residual capacity.

Mean Arterial Blood Pressure

MABP was recorded from an indwelling arterial catheter in all infants.

Cerebro-Electrical Activity

aEEG was monitored continuously from biparietal electrodes using a cerebral function monitor (CFM, Critikon, Tampa, Fla., USA) from 1 h before until 2 h after the surfactant instillation.

Cerebral Oxygenation and Cerebral Blood Volume

CBV and cerebral oxyhaemoglobin (HbO_2) were monitored with NIRS continuously for half an hour before administration of surfactant and for 1 h after. Details of the NIRS system have been described elsewhere [12]. Our NIRS instrument (Radiometer, Copenhagen, Denmark) uses four semiconductor laser diodes with wavelengths of 775, 805, 845 and 904 nm. Using NIRS it is possible to calculate changes in HbO_2, deoxyhaemoglobin concentration and total haemoglobin concentration. When the optical path length is known it is possible to calculate the total CBV. In these studies we have used the assumption that the optical light path length is 4.39 times the interoptode distance [13].

Cerebral Blood Flow

CBF was measured 15 min before and 5 and 60 min after administration of surfactant. ^{133}Xe (20–40 MBq/kg) was injected into a peripheral vein, and the clearance was recorded by two scintillation detectors placed over one frontoparietal region and the thorax, respectively. CBF was calculated from the time the activity of xenon in the lung had decreased to 15% of its peak activity [14].

Ethical Aspects

The study was approved by the Ethical Committee of Copenhagen and Frederiksberg. The infants were enrolled in the study after informed consent by their parents.

Statistics

Values below are given as mean ± SD, or mean and 95% confidence intervals (CI_{95}).

Results

Clinical Response

Arterial/alveolar oxygen tension ratio ($PaO_2/FiO_2 \times 0.95 - PaCO_2$) before treatment and 15 min after treatment averaged 0.11 ± 0.05 and 0.34 ± 0.17 ($p < 0.001$),

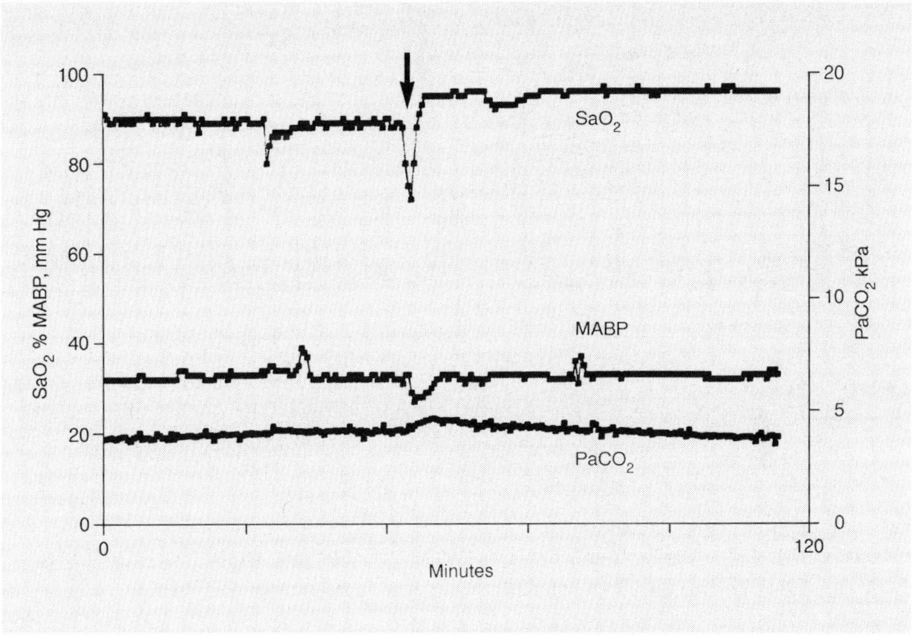

Fig. 1. Change in arterial oxygen saturation (SaO_2; upper curve), mean arterial blood pressure (MABP; middle curve) and $PaCO_2$ (lower curve) during and following surfactant administration (indicated by arrow).

respectively. There was a reduction in oxygen requirement (FiO_2) after 15 min in all but 4 babies. Three infants had IVH grade 1–11 before surfactant treatment. Five infants ultimately developed an IVH grade I–II and 8 grade III–IV [15]. Twelve of the 34 infants died (35%).

Oesophageal and Central Venous Pressure

OP or CVP measured in 10 infants increased slightly but not significantly during surfactant administration (mean values before and 5 min after treatment: 2.8 and 3.4 mm Hg, respectively; $p = 0.54$).

Mean Arterial Blood Pressure

The maximal fall in MABP averaged –9 mm Hg (CI_{95} –11 to –6 mm Hg), and this occurred within 1–2 min after surfactant instillation. The decrease after 5 min was much smaller (mean –2.8 mm Hg; $p = 0.05$). MABP returned to the pretreatment level by 15 min after surfactant administration in the majority of patients (fig. 1).

Arterial Oxygen Saturation

Arterial oxygen saturation (SaO_2) measured by pulse oximetry decreased markedly (mean –9.5%; CI_{95} –11.8 to –7.2%) during the 30–60 s of surfactant administration, which followed by a large increase in SaO_2 (mean 8.1%; CI_{95} 4.6 to 11.5%). The initial fall in saturation was not significantly different from the decrease observed in 16 babies during endotracheal tube suctioning prior to surfactant instillation (mean –8.3; CI_{95} –10.0 to –6.1%).

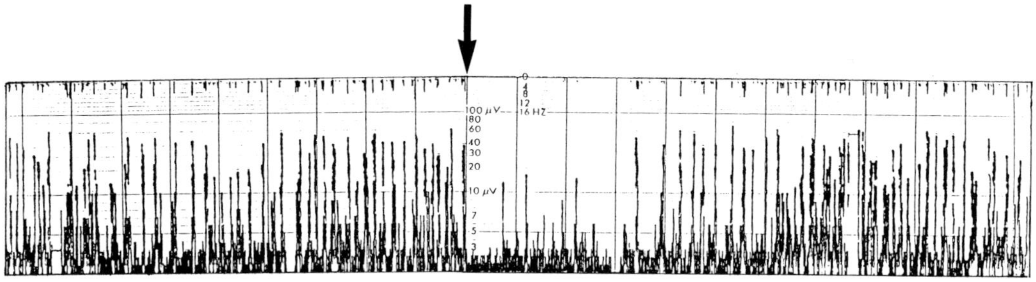

Fig. 2. Cerebral function monitor recording during surfactant instillation (indicated by arrow).

EEG

A decrease in the EEG burst rate was seen in all but 2 infants for a period of 10–20 min after administration of surfactant (fig. 2). There were no differences in the CFM patterns of babies developing IVH and those without IVH, nor between those given surfactant before or after 12 h of postnatal age. No correlation was found between the decrease in burst rate (within the first 10 min) and the magnitude of the fall in MABP. Endotracheal suctioning was not associated with any changes in aEEG activity.

Cerebral Oxygenation and Cerebral Blood Volume

Cerebral HbO_2 concentration decreased slightly during surfactant administration in parallel to the fall in SaO_2 but this was followed by a large increase (mean 0.15 mmol/l·cm; CI_{95} 0.10 to 0.20 mmol/l·cm. However, the reduction in oxyhaemoglobin was not greater than the reduction which occurred during endotracheal suctioning. A rise in CBV lasting for 10–15 min (mean 0.12 ml/100 g; CI_{95} 0.03–0.21 ml/100 g) was seen in 19 of 21 infants studied with NIRS (fig. 3). The rise in CBV was equivalent to the response of the cerebral circulation to a 2-kPa increase in $PaCO_2$ [13]. After 60 min, CBV had decreased below the pretreatment level. The decrease paralleled a decrease in $PaCO_2$ [4].

Cerebral Blood Flow

CBF before treatment averaged 14.5 ± 5.9 ml/100 g·min and rose slightly but nor significantly in the recording obtained just after surfactant administration (mean 15.1 ± 5.4 ml/100 g·min). One hour after surfactant administration there was a decrease in mean CBF to 11.9 ml/100 g·min ($p < 0.05$), which paralleled the decrease in $PaCO_2$.

Discussion

A transient but clear depression in EEG activity after administration of surfactant to preterm babies has previously been demonstrated, concurrent with a reduced arterial O_2 content and a fall in arterial blood pressure [3, 4]. We hypothesised therefore that cerebral ischaemia could account for the EEG depression. Using NIRS, we demonstrated a brief period of cerebral hypoxia after surfactant

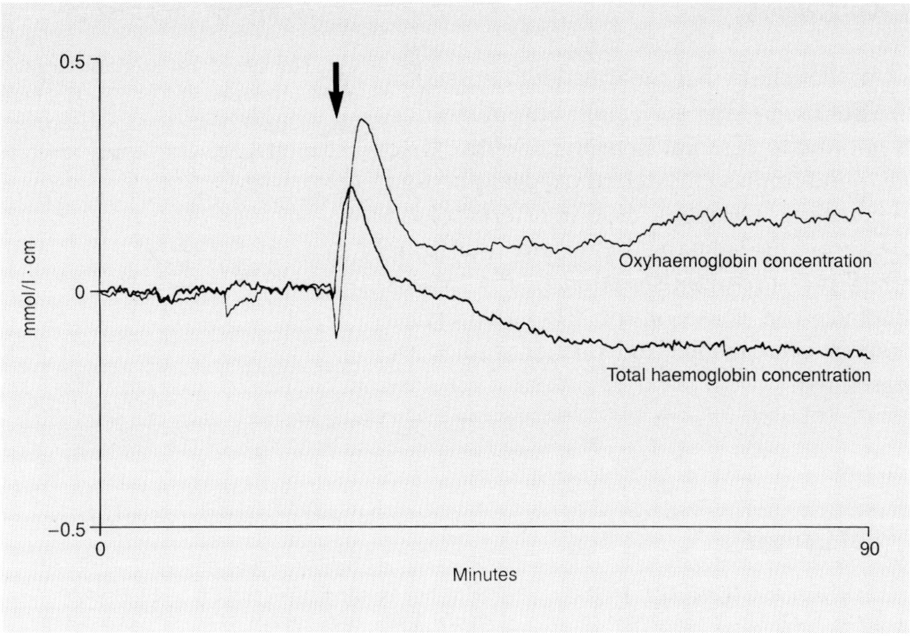

Fig. 3. Change in concentration of oxyhaemoglobin and total haemoglobin during surfactant administration (indicated by arrow).

administration, with a fall in HbO_2 concurrent with a fall in SaO_2 followed by an increase in cerebral oxygenation. The transient falls in oxyhaemoglobin and oxygen saturation were similar to those seen during endotracheal suctioning when changes in EEG are not observed. Concurrent with the fall in HbO_2, a rise in CBV was observed which may have been as a compensatory response to hypoxia. These NIRS findings have been confirmed recently by Edwards et al. [5], although another study showed no change in CBV after surfactant treatment [6].

Changes in CBV and CBF are usually proportional. It is possible, however, that CBF may decrease in the presence of an increased CBV as a result of venous stasis. Our measurement of CVP and OP makes such an explanation for the observed increase in CBV unlikely. Furthermore, the study of CBF using ^{133}Xe clearance demonstrated unchanged CBF during 15 min following surfactant therapy. This is consistent with the NIRS results as ^{133}Xe clearance is measured over 15 min and a transient increase is not excluded.

Studies of cerebral blood flow velocity (CBFV) after surfactant administration using Doppler technique have yielded conflicting results with increased [7], unchanged [8, 11] or decreased [9, 10] CBFV. These differences may be due to the timing of the measurements. Furthermore, there is an inherent uncertainty about the relation between CBFV and CBF due to insonating vessels which may constrict or dilate as part of the cerebrovascular response.

Conclusion

We conclude that the transient depression in aEEG seen after surfactant administration is not due to cerebral ischaemia. With NIRS we found improved cerebral oxygenation and hyperaemia. Despite a drop in arterial blood pressure, CBF remained constant indicating intact pressure-autoregulation in the infants studied. The cause of the EEG depression remains unexplained and further studies are warranted.

Acknowledgements

The surfactant used in the present trial (Curosurf) was developed by Tore Curstedt and Bengt Robertson, Stockholm, with financial support from the Swedish Medical Research Council (Project 3351) and II:s Jubileumsfond.

References

1 Collaborative European Multicenter Study Group: Surfactant replacement therapy for severe neonatal respiratory distress syndrome: An international randomized clinical trial. Pediatrics 1988;82:683–691.

2 Robertson B: Neonatal respiratory distress syndrome and surfactant therapy: A brief review. Eur Respir J 1989;2(suppl 3):73–76.

3 Skov L, Hellström-Westas L, Jacobsen T, Greisen G, Svenningsen NW: Acute changes in cerebral oxygenation and cerebral blood volume in preterm infants during surfactant treatment. Neuropediatrics, in press.

4 Hellström-Westas L, Bell AH, Skov L, Greisen G, Svenningsen NW: Cerebro-electrical depression following surfactant treatment in preterm neonates. Pediatrics, in press.

5 Edwards AD, McCormick DC, Roth SC, Wyatt JS, Cope M, Delpy DT, Reynolds EOR: Effects of porcine surfactant (Curosurf) on the cerebral oxygenation and haemodynamics in preterm infants (abstract) Zürich, ESPR, 1991, p 199.

6 Fahnenstich H: Near infrared spectroscopy – relative changes in cerebral hemodynamics under surfactant therapy. Biol Neonate 1991;59:388.

7 Van de Bor M, Ma EJ, Walther FJ: Cerebral blood flow velocity after surfactant instillation in preterm infants. J Pediatrics 1991;118:285–287.

8 Jorch G, Rabe H, Garbe M, Michel E, Gortner L: Acute and protracted effects of intratracheal surfactant application on internal carotid blood flow velocity, blood pressure and carbondioxide tension in very low birth weight infants. Eur J Pediatr 1989;148:770–773.

9 Hascoët JM, Hamon I, Santos E, Legagneur M, Monin P, Vert P: Effect of surfactant on cerebral circulation (abstract). Zürich, ESPR, 1991, p 200.

10 Cowan F, Silverman M, Wertheim D, Whitelaw A: The acute effects of surfactant administration on blood pressure and cerebral blood flow velocity in the neonate (abstract); in Speer CP, Robertson B (eds): Proceedings of the 4th Workshop on Surfactant-Replacement, Göttingen, 1989, p 14.

11 McCord B, Halliday HL, McClure G, Reid MMcC: Changes in pulmonary and cerebral blood flow after surfactant treatment for severe respiratory distress syndrome; in Lachmann B (ed): Surfactant Replacement Therapy in Neonatal and Adult Respiratory Distress Syndrome. Berlin, Springer, 1989, pp 195–200.

12 Pryds P, Greisen G, Skov L, Friis-Hansen B: Carbon dioxide related changes in cerebral blood volume and cerebral blood flow in mechanically ventilated, preterm neonates: Comparison of near infrared spectrophotometry and ^{133}Xenon clearance. Pediatr Res 1990;27:445–449.

13 Wray S, Cope M, Delpy DT, Wyatt JS, Reynolds EOR: Characterization of the near infrared absorption spectra of cytochrome aa_3 and haemoglobin for the non-invasive monitoring of cerebral oxygenation. Biochim Biophys Acta 1988;933:184–192.

14 Greisen G: Cerebral blood flow in mechanically ventilated, preterm neonates. Dan Med Bull 1990;2:124–132.

15 Papile L, Burstein J, Burstein R, Koffler H: Incidence and evolution of subependymal and intraventricular hemorrhage: A study of infants with birth weights less than 1500 gm. J Pediatr 1978;92:529–534.

Original Paper

Biol Neonate 1992;61(suppl 1):37–43

Dominique Haumont[a]
Claudia Rössle[b]
Anne Clercx[a]
Marianne Spehl[a]
Armand Biver[a]
Myriam Richelle[b]
Yvon A. Carpentier[b]

Departments of
[a] Pediatrics and
[b] Clinical Nutrition,
Free University of Brussels,
Belgium

Modifications of Surfactant Phospholipid Pattern in Premature Infants Treated with Curosurf: Clinical and Dietary Correlations

Key Words
Pulmonary surfactants
Respiratory distress syndrome
Phospholipids
Intravenous fat emulsions

Abstract
Neonatal respiratory distress syndrome (RDS) is characterized by an immature surfactant phospholipid pattern. We aimed to study the evolution of surfactant phospholipids over a 6-day period, before and after surfactant replacement therapy with Curosurf, and to investigate possible interactions with exogenous phospholipids administered during total parenteral nutrition (TPN). Seventeen premature infants with RDS were randomly assigned to receive TPN with lipids or without (glucose group). Both groups showed a similar evolution of the surfactant phospholipids. At day 6, the surfactant composition had changed towards a mature human surfactant pattern except for phosphatidylglycerol which remained low (1%), compensated for by a high phosphatidylinositol and phosphatidylserine proportion (13.3%), Phospholipid subcomponents in plasma remained unchanged in both groups. Plasma total cholesterol (151 ± 18 vs. 113 ± 6 mg/dl, $p < 0.05$) and cholesteryl esters (172 ± 20 vs. 113 ± 9 mg/dl, $p < 0.01$) were higher in the glucose than in the lipid group. Total calorie intake was significantly higher in the lipid group (85 ± 4 vs. 64 ± 6 kcal/kg·day, $p < 0.01$).

Introduction

Replacement therapy with porcine surfactant (Curosurf) has been shown to improve lung function and short-term outcome in premature infants with severe respiratory distress syndrome (RDS) [1]. Until now, the role of the different lipids present in the exogenous surfactant and their interactions with endogenous surfactant have received little at-

Dominique Haumont
Neonatal Unit
Saint-Pierre University Hospital
rue Haute 322
B-1000 Brussels (Belgium)

0006–3126/92/
0617–0037$2.75/0

tention. Measurements of the different phospholipid subcomponents such as phosphatidylcholine (PC), sphingomyelin (SM), phosphatidylglycerol (PG), phosphatidylinositol (PI), phosphatidylethanolamine (PE) and phosphatidylserine (PS) have been used to predict fetal lung maturity [2]. Phospholipid composition of lung effluent in preterm infants before and after treatment with human surfactant has been documented by Hallman et al. [3] but has not been studied in preterm infants treated with other surfactants. Curosurf contains approximately 99% polar lipids, mainly phospholipids and 1% hydrophobic proteins (SPB and SPC). Structural and functional characteristics have been published [4].

Early administration of intravenous lipids is still a matter of debate and not unanimously accepted. While delaying lipid supply has been reported to adversely influence both essential fatty acid pattern (EFA) [5] and surfactant composition [6], other authors associated increased respiratory difficulty with early intravenous lipid administration [7].

In the present study, we evaluated surfactant composition and ventilatory requirements in preterm infants with RDS treated with Curosurf and randomized to receive lipid-containing or lipid-free total parenteral nutrition (TPN).

Material and Methods

Patient Selection

Seventeen premature infants were prospectively enrolled to receive surfactant rescue treatment at the neonatal Units of the 'Hôpital Universitaire Saint-Pierre' or the 'Hôpital Universitaire des Enfants Reine Fabiola', Brussels, Belgium. Eligibility criteria were. (1) gestational age <35 weeks; (2) clinical and radiological findings typical of neonatal RDS; (3) age when treated: 2–24 h; (4) requirement of artificial ventilation; (5) $FiO_2 > 0.6$; (6) presence of an arterial catheter; (7) no complicating disease; (8) informed parental consent. Exclusion criteria were: (1) major congenital malformations; (2) surgical condition; (3) maternal drug abuse.

The protocol had been approved by the ethical committee of the two hospitals.

Surfactant Treatment and Ventilator Settings

Three batches of porcine surfactant (Curosurf, Chiesi, Parma, Italy) were used in the trial (table 1). A first dose of 200 mg/kg was administered in all babies before the age of 24 h. A second dose of 100 mg/kg was allowed 6–18 h later if ventilatory requirements and FiO_2 increased. The surfactant was administered into each main bronchus with a sterile feeding catheter. Ventilator settings were adjusted by the attending neonatologists according to transcutaneous blood gas monitoring, arterial blood sampling and clinical response. Ventilatory Index (VI) was calculated as mean airway pressure $\times$ FiO_2/PaO_2 cm H_2O/mm Hg.

Randomisation

Infants were randomised once surfactant eligibility criteria were met. They were assigned to TPN regimen with lipids (lipid group) or without (glucose group). Characteristics of both groups are given in table 2.

Parenteral Nutrition

The two TPN regimens were as follows: the glucose group received amino acids up to 2.5 g/kg·day and glucose up to 10–18 g/kg·day; the lipid group received amino acids up to 2.5 g/kg·day, glucose up to 11–17 g/kg·day and lipids, stepwise up to 2–3 g triglycerides/kg·day. Lipids were supplemented as a 20% soybean emulsion, emulsified with egg-yolk phospholipids (Lipovenös 20%, Fresenius AG, Bad Homburg, FRG). The phospholipid composition of the emulsion is given in table 2. The regimens were meant to be isocaloric, inasmuch as glucose intake was not limited by individual glucose tolerance. Administration of vitamins, electrolytes and trace elements was similar in both groups.

Sampling

Tracheal aspirates were obtained during routine suctioning and any fluid obtained was collected in a Leuken's trap and kept at 4 °C. Since preterm infants with RDS have very little surfactant to be aspirated, all samples were pooled until surfactant treatment was administered. These samples are referred to as 'pretreatment'. Sampling was also performed at 24 h and again at 6 days after treatment. Pharyngeal aspirates obtained at birth in 11 healthy term newborns provided reference values for mature human surfactant

Table 1. Phospholipid subcomponent distribution in Curosurf and the lipid emulsion compared to mature human surfactant (% of total phospholipids)

Phospholipid subcomponents	Curosurf %	Emulsion %	Mature human surfactant, %
Phosphatidylcholine	66.8±2.9	80.8	76.3±2.0
Sphingomyelin	9.2±0.9	2.1	1.3±0.3
Phosphatidylinositol + phosphatidylserine	5.8±1.4	0.1	7.3±1.7
Phosphatidylglycerol	2.5±0.06		7.3±0.7
Phosphatidylethanolamine	11.7±3.0	12.0	5.0±0.9
Lysophosphatidylcholine	2.8±2.8	5.1	0.8±0.2
Others	1.05±0.32		2.7±0.5

Values are given as mean ± SEM.

Table 2. Characteristics of study infants

Parameters	Lipid group (n = 9)	Glucose group (n = 8)
Birthweight, g	1,448±145	1,730±267
Gestational age, weeks	30.3±0.8	30.5±1.1
Sex male	7	7
female	2	1
Age at Curosurf instillation, h	6 (3.5–12)	6 (4–17)
FiO_2, pretreatment	0.87±0.05	0.83±0.05
VI, pretreatment	0.20±0.03	0.19±0.03

Values are given as mean ± SEM or median (range).
VI = Ventilatory Index.

(table 1). Three milliliters of blood was sampled before surfactant treatment (day 0) and again at day 6.

Sample Treatment

The aspirates were gently homogenized and centrifuged at 150 *g* for 5 min to remove cell debris. The supernatant was recentrifuged at 7,500 *g* for 40 min if the volume exceeded 0.5 ml. The resulting surfactant pellet was then resuspended in 0.5 ml of 0.15 *M* NaCl and kept at –80 °C until analysis.

Blood samples were collected in disodiumethylendiamine-tetraacetic acid (EDTA) containing glass tubes and centrifuged, and plasma was kept at –80 °C until analysis.

Chemical Analyses

The plasma concentrations of total triglycerides (TG), total cholesterol (TC), free cholesterol (FC) and nonesterified fatty acids (NEFAs) were determined by means of enzymatic-colorimetric tests using available kits (Test-Combination Triglycerides without free glycerol, Monotest cholesterol CHOD-PAP, Test-combination free cholesterol (Boehringer, Mannheim, FRG), and NEFA QUICK 'BMY' (Boehringer Mannheim & Yamanouchi KK, Tokyo, Japan).

Total phosphorus concentrations in suspensions of tracheal aspirates and plasma were determined according to Bartlett [8]. Aliquots of the samples containing 200–300 nmol total phosphorus were extracted with 20 vol of chloroform/methanol (2:1, v/v) [9]. After addition of 0.2 vol of 0.1 *M* KCl, the clear chloroform phase was evaporated at 40 °C under nitrogen. The residue was redissolved in 20–40 µl of chloroform/methanol (2:1, v/v) and the phospholipid subclasses were separated by two-dimensional thin-layer chromatography using 20 × 20 cm TLC plates precoated with 0.25 mm silicagel 60 (Merck, Darmstadt, FRG). A slight modification of the solvent systems from Casals et al. [10] was used. The solvent for the first dimension was chloroform/methanol/water (70:26:3.5, v/v), and the solvent for the second dimension was chloroform/methanol/acetic acid/H_2O (84.5:34:9.8:2.2, v/v). Spots were visualized with iodine vapour and the individual phospholipids identified by comparison to a mixture of reference phospholipids (all from Sigma, St. Louis, Mo., USA).

The areas containing the different phospholipids were scraped into acid-rinsed glass tubes and phospholipids were eluted by rinsing 3 times with 2 ml chloroform/methanol 2:1 (v/v). Spots of PI and PS usually were not well separated and, therefore, scraped together. The amount of organic phosphorus was determined [8] and the results for each phospholipid given in % of total phosphorus measured in all scraped spots.

Statistical Analyses

Differences between groups were analysed by means of unpaired t test. Evolution within groups was assessed with the paired t test.

Table 3. Clinical outcome characteristics

Parameters	Lipid group (n = 9)	Glucose group (n = 7)
IVH grade III–IV	2	1
Day of extubation	8 (1–58)	7 (4–25)
Age at weaning from O_2, days	7 (1–64)	13 (4–31)
PTX	1	2
BPD scoring	2 (1–8)	3 (1–6)

Values are given as median (range).

IVH = Intraventricular hemorrhage, BPD = bronchopulmonary dysplasia, scored from chest films by one of us (M.S.) according to Toce et al. [11].

Results

Clinical Outcome

Ventilatory requirements significantly dropped over the 6-day period and tended to be lower in the lipid group compared to the glucose group (average FiO_2 0.24 and 0.28, and average ventilatory index 0.019 and 0.031, respectively; NS). The total calorie intake at day 6 was significantly lower in the glucose group (64 vs. 85 kcal/kg·day, $p < 0.01$). The overall clinical outcome was very heterogenous in the two groups (table 3). Sixteen of the 17 patients survived and were discharged without O_2 treatment.

Evolution of Surfactant Phospholipid Pattern in Tracheal Aspirates

The distribution of individual phospholipids in the alveolar lining fluid is shown in figure 1. Before surfactant treatment a classical immature phospholipid pattern was observed, characterised by relatively low PC concentration (< 60%), high SM and low PG. No difference was observed between lipid and glucose groups. Twenty-four hours after Curosurf instillation, the phospholipid pattern of aspirates showed an increase of PC above 60%, with other phospholipid subcomponents being found almost in the same proportion as in Curosurf. After 6 days, analysis was performed in 14 infants: one patient from the glucose group had died of severe neurological damage, and 2 patients from the lipid group had been extubated.

The phospholipid pattern at day 6 is given in figure 1. The proportion of PC showed a further increase (73% in the glucose group and 76% in the lipid group) and was comparable to that found in mature human surfactant (76%). The relative concentration of PG, one of the classical markers of lung maturity, remained at a much lower level than in mature human surfactant (1 vs. 7.3%). The high

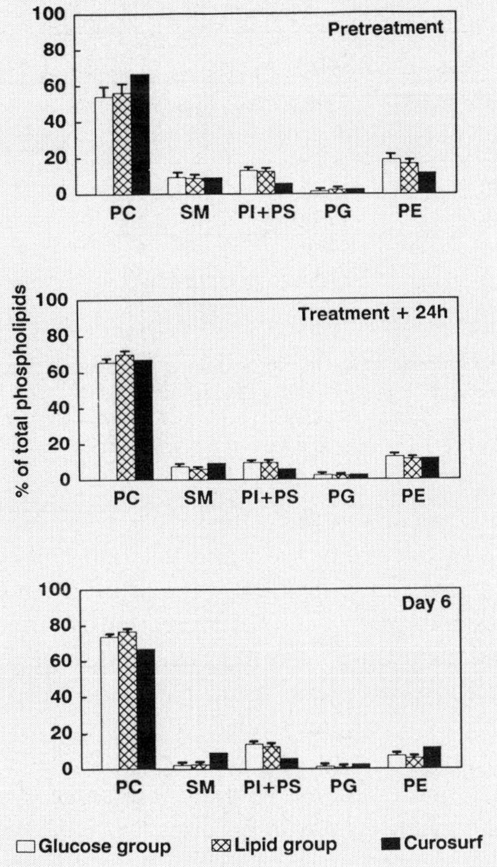

1

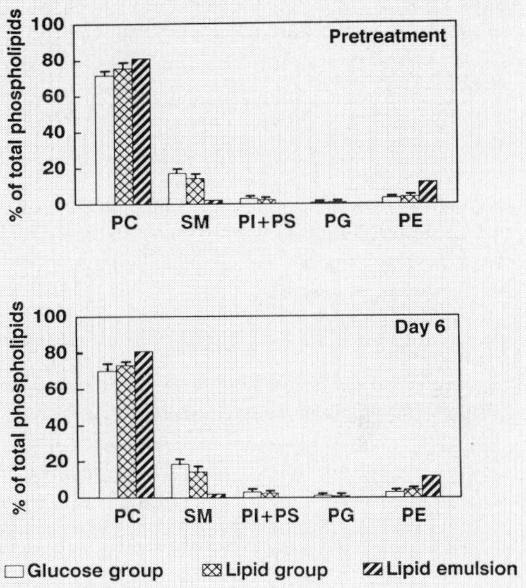

2

Fig. 1. Phospholipid pattern in tracheal aspirates obtained before Curosurf treatment, 24 h after instillation of Curosurf and at day 6. Results are given for the 2 groups of patients and compared to the composition of Curosurf phospholipid pattern. Abbreviations are explained in the text.

Fig. 2. Phospholipid pattern in the plasma before Curosurf treatment and at day 6. Results are given for the 2 groups of patients and compared to the phospholipid composition of the lipid emulsion.

proportion of PE and SM in the immature surfactant decreased significantly after 6 days in both groups ($p < 0.001$).

Evolution of Plasma Lipids

The glucose group which did not receive any lipid intake over the 6-day period showed a phospholipid pattern similar to the other group who received up to 120 mg phospholipids/kg·day (fig. 2). Triglycerides remained at low levels in both groups suggesting an efficient clearance of the emulsion in the lipid group (table 4). Phospholipids and NEFAs were also similar. Concentrations of total cholesterol and cholesteryl esters were significantly higher in the glucose group.

Discussion

The present study demonstrates that exogenous porcine surfactant (Curosurf) instillated in preterm infants with RDS induces substantial modifications of the characteristic immature human surfactant phospholipid pattern over time. The measurements per-

Table 4. Plasma lipid concentrations obtained before Curosurf treatment and at day 6 in the two TPN groups

	Pretreatment		Day 6		
	lipid group (n = 9)	glucose group (n = 8)	lipid group (n = 9)	glucose group (n = 7)	p
Triglycerides, mg/dl	43±9	23±3	52±8	48±7	
Total cholesterol, mg/dl	61±9	60±4	113±6	151±18	<0.05
Free cholesterol, mg/dl	19±2	21±2	46±3	49±6	
Cholesteryl esters, mg/dl	72±14	65±5	113±9	172±20	<0.01
Phospholipids, mg/dl	93±8	118±6	220±14	207±17	
NEFAs, μmol/l	127±35	78±14	81±10	59±11	

Values are given as mean ± SEM.

formed at day 6 showed a surfactant pattern resembling but not like mature human surfactant. PC concentration was increased and SM decreased but the main difference consisted in the persistence of low PG an high PS+PI contents. Although PG is considered a biological marker of mature human surfactant [2], its role regarding tensioactive properties is not confirmed by our results. This is in agreement with studies in term newborn rabbits, where Hallmann et al. [12] observed no sign of RDS even though surfactant contained little PG. In addition, Beppu et al. [13] demonstrated no lung function impairment in adult rabbits, in which surfactant was made PG deficient by administration of inositol. In these animal studies, PG deficiency was counterbalanced by an increase in PI. This was also observed in the present work. It has been suggested that PI could act as an effective substitute for PG in adults. Whether this could be extrapolated to preterm infants receiving porcine surfactant treatment remains speculative. On the other hand, King et al. [14] have shown that PG plays an important role in the interaction between surfactant apoproteins and phospholipids.

In this study, we could not find any biochemical modification of the SPLP when exogenous phospholipids were infused in the bloodstream as a component of lipid emulsion. Nevertheless, the neonates who received intravenous lipids tended to have lower ventilatory requirement after 6 days. Long-term outcomes were too heterogenous and did not allow conclusions to be drawn. It is obvious that the clinical outcome is dependent on so many factors for each individual baby. An interesting difference between both groups was the higher concentration of total cholesterol due to increased cholesteryl esters in the glucose group. In another part of the study [unpubl.], we analyzed the individual fatty acids esterifying cholesterol. Cholesterol esterification can take place in the circulation catalysed by lecithin:cholesterolacyltransferase (LCAT) or in the cells mediated by acyl:cholesterolacyltransferase (ACAT). LCAT preferentially transfers polyunsaturated essential fatty acids, whereas ACAT transfers non essential fatty acids. Cholesterol in the glucose group was predominantly esterified with saturated and mono-unsaturated fatty acids (palmitoleate, palmitate and oleate) whereas in the lipid group cholesteryl esters contained larger amounts of polyunsaturated fatty acids (mainly linoleate). The fatty acid pattern of cholesteryl esters in the glucose group may indicate an enhanced activity of intracellular ACAT. However, a further impairment of LCAT activity which is already low in preterm infants cannot be excluded [15]. The role of LCAT may be important in providing lysophosphatidylcholines to tissues for new lecithin synthesis [15, 16].

From the data of the present study we conclude that, in preterm infants receiving Curosurf, the immature surfactant phospholipid pattern is modified towards a pattern closer to mature human surfactant but with a low relative concentration of PG. Exogenous phospholipids included in lipid emulsions do not influence the surfactant phospholipid pattern over a 6 day period. However, lipid-containing TPN allows a higher calorie intake and provides C:18 essential fatty acids of n–6 and n–3 families. Increasing total calorie intake was difficult when no lipids were added to the regimen.

Acknowledgment

The authors thank Dr. B. Robertson, director of the Curosurf trials, for his continuous support, and Dr. A. Dachy and Dr. H.L. Vis for their encouragement. We also thank Mrs. P. D'Hondt for the skillful technical assistance and the nurses of both neonatal units for collecting the tracheal aspirates, and express our gratitude to Miss N. Van Laer for typing the manuscript.

References

1 Collaborative European Multicenter Study Group: Surfactant replacement therapy for severe neonatal respiratory distress syndrome: An international randomised clinical trial. Pediatrics 1988;82:683–691.

2 Hallman M: Antenatal diagnosis of lung maturity; in Robertson B, Van Golde LMG, Batenburg JJ (eds): Pulmonary Surfactant. Elsevier, Amsterdam, 1984, pp 419–448.

3 Hallman M, Merritt AT, Pohjavuori M, Gluck L: Effect of surfactant substitution on long effluent phospholipids in respiratory distress syndrome: Evaluation of surfactant phospholipid turnover, pool size, and the relationship to severity of respiratory failure. Pediatr Res 1986;20:1228–1235.

4 Robertson B, Curstedt T, Johansson Y, Jörnvall H, Kobayashi T: Structural and functional characterization of porcine surfactant isolated by lipid-gel-chromatography. Prog Respir Res 1989;25:237–246.

5 Farrell PM: Essential fatty acid deficiency in premature infants. Am J Clin Nutr 1988;48:220–229.

6 Friedman Z, Rosenberg A: Abnormal lung surfactant related to essential fatty acid deficiency in the neonate. Pediatrics 1979;63:855–859.

7 Hammerman C, Aramburo MJ: Decreased lipid intake reduces morbidity in sick premature neonates. J Pediatr 1988;113:1083–1088.

8 Bartlett GR: Phosphorus assay in column chromatography. J Biol Chem 1959;234:466–468.

9 Folch J, Lees M, Sloane Stanley GH: A simple method for the isolation and purification of total lipids from animal tissue. J Biol Chem 1957; 226:497–509.

10 Casals C, Herrera L, Mighel E, Garcia-Barrerre P, Municio AM: Comparison between intra- and extracellular surfactant in respiratory distress induced by oleic acid. Biochim Biophys Acta 1989;1003:201–203.

11 Toce SS, Farrell PM, Leavitt LA, Samuels DP, Edwards DK: Clinical and roentgenographic scoring systems for assessing bronchopulmonary dysplasia. Am J Dis Child 1984;138:581–585.

12 Hallman M, Gluck L: Phosphatidylglycerol in lung surfactant. III. Possible modifier of surfactant function. J Lipid Res 1976;17:257–262.

13 Beppu OS, Clements JA, Goerke J: Phosphatidylglycerol deficient lung surfactant has normal properties. J Appl Physiol 1983;55:496–502.

14 King RJ, Macbeth MC: Interaction of the lipid and protein components of pulmonary surfactant. Role of phosphatidylglycerol and calcium. Biochim Biophys Acta 1981;647: 159–168.

15 Papadopoulos A, Hamosh M, Chowdry P, Scanlon JW, Hamosh P: Lecithin-cholesterol acyltransferase in newborn infants: low activity levels in preterm infants. J Pediatr 1988;113:896–898.

16 Stein Y, Stein O: Metabolism of labeled lysolecithin, lysophosphatidylethanolamine and lecithin in the rat. Biochim Biophys Acta 1966; 116:95–107.

Original Paper

Biol Neonate 1992;61(suppl 1):44–47

Nils W. Svenningsen
Lars Björklund
Carsten Vilstrup
Olof Werner

Neonatal Intensive Care Unit, Departments of Paediatrics and Anaesthesiology, University Hospital, Lund, Sweden

Lung Mechanics (FRC and Static Pressure-Volume Diagram) after Endotracheal Surfactant Instillation: Preliminary Observations

Key Words
Lung compliance
Functional residual capacity
Pulmonary surfactants
Respiratory distress syndrome

Abstract
Preliminary measurements of functional residual capacity (FRC) with the sulphurhexafluoride technique and static pressure volume diagrams were performed in newborn infants with respiratory distress syndrome receiving endotracheal instillation of natural porcine surfactant (Curosurf, 100 or 200 mg/kg). Within the first hour after surfactant treatment there was an increase in FRC and distensibility of the lungs persisting for 24–48 h.

Prospective randomized controlled studies have shown that endotracheal administration of surfactant improves oxygenation as gas exchange in babies with neonatal respiratory distress syndrome RDS [1]. Endotracheal surfactant instillation also improves lung mechanics in immature neonatal lambs [2]. The aim of the present studies is to evaluate lung mechanics and volumes immediately before and after surfactant instillation in ventilated babies with respiratory distress syndrome (RDS).

Methods

Functional residual capacity (FRC) was measured by a computerized multiple breath washout technique using the inert tracer gas sulphurhexafluoride (SF-6) [3]. During washout, the volume of SF-6 was calculated by a computer every 10 ms from signals representing expiratory flow and SF-6 concentrations measured by a fast infrared analyser. These measurement procedures are highly automated and the results are directly presented online by the computer immediately after the washout. In model lung tests with the SF-6 technique accurate and reproducible results were obtained [4].

For the static pressure-volume diagram measurements, we used a computerized interrupter technique [5]. Muscle relaxants are required and it is necessary to

Nils W. Svenningsen
Department of Paediatrics
University Hospital
S-221 85 Lund (Sweden)

0006–3126/92/
0617–0044$2.75/0

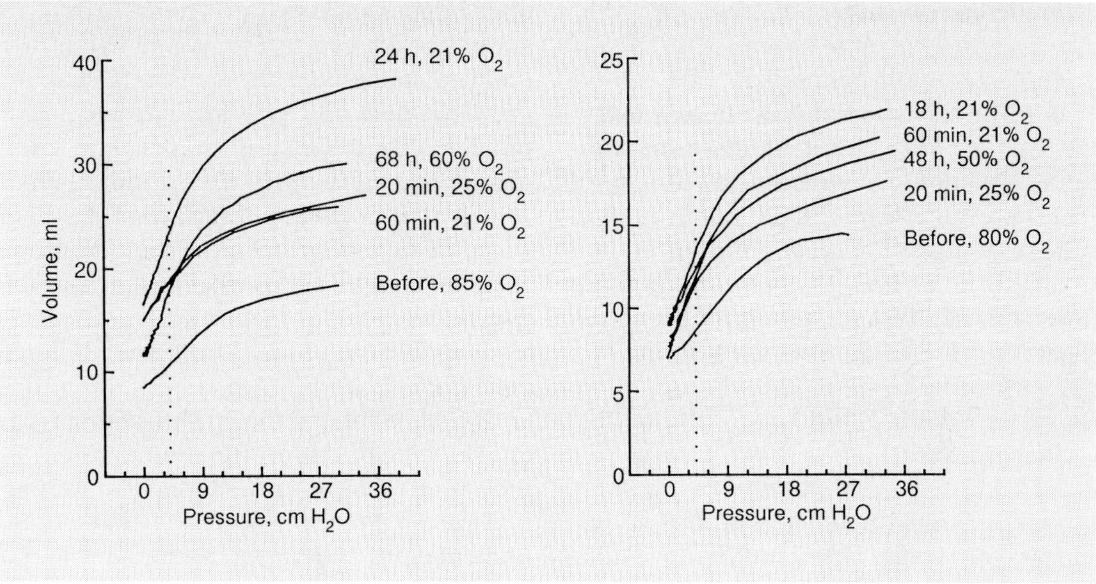

Fig. 1. P/V curves in preterm infants with RDS (left panel, boy, birthweight 1,250 g, gestational age 31 weeks; right panel, girl, birthweight 930 g, gestational age 28 weeks) illustrating changes in lung distensibility and decrease in oxygen requirement after a single dose of Curosurf (200 mg/kg) given by endotracheal instillation. The vertical stippled line indicates the positive end-expiratory pressure which was kept constant at 4 cm H_2O. The increasing volumes along this line indicate the rapid rise in FRC after surfactant instillation.

occlude the airway around the tube if any leaks are present. After inflation of the lung to 30 cm H_2O the baby expires passively and the expiratory flow is interrupted by an automatically occluding valve for 80 ms every 160 ms. An on-line pneumotachograph and pressure transducer register the volume and airway pressure and the computer draws the static pressure-volume curve.

The infants were treated with a Servo ventilator 900 C and monitored continuously with a heart rate monitor and a transcutaneous pO_2 and pCO_2 monitor (Tina, Radiometer A/S Copenhagen, Denmark).

The natural porcine surfactant preparation (Curosurf) was given in a dose of 100 or 200 mg/kg either as a single dose or divided in two separate boluses into each lung. The baby was in the supine position and was rotated 30° right or left when receiving the surfactant in divided doses. After instillation the baby was manually ventilated for 20–30 s before being reconnected to the ventilator.

Patients

The patient group comprised 8 preterm infants with RDS treated in the neonatal intensive care unit at Lund University Hospital. The inclusion criteria for surfactant instillation were clinical and radiological evidence of RDS and the need for endotracheal intubation for ventilation and $FiO_2 > 0.40$. The range of gestational age was 26–32 weeks (mean 28 weeks) and of birthweight 830–1,860 g (mean 1,100 g). The postnatal age at surfactant treatment ranged from 2 to 18 h (mean 6 h).

Informed parental consent was obtained in all cases and the study was approved by the Ethical Committee of Lund University.

Preliminary Results

Our data are still preliminary. FRC at 4 cm H_2O PEEP increased in most infants within the first hour after surfactant treatment. Maximum deflation compliance showed a rapid increase within 20 min in all infants as illustrated in figure 1. Maximum effect was usually seen around 18–24 h after a single dose of Curosurf, and at 48 h FRC was still higher than before Curosurf instillation.

Discussion

Only a limited number of studies of pulmonary mechanics after surfactant instillation in preterm newborn infants have been published [6–9]. One study showed improvement in tidal minute volume and dynamic compliance after bovine surfactant instillation during spontaneous respiration but not during mechanical ventilation [6]. Another study found no significant changes in dynamic compliance until 24 h after surfactant instillation [7]. A recent report on the effect of rescue doses of artificial surfactant (Exosurf) showed improvement in respiratory system static compliance only 1 week after surfactant instillation [8]. These studies failed to show any change in lung mechanics during the first hours after surfactant treatment. However, recently Edberg et al. [9] studied the effects of instillation of human surfactant in 4 preterm infants with severe RDS during mechanical ventilation using a body plethysmograph and a modified nitrogen washout method. These authors found an immediate rise in lung volume with an increase in FRC of 20–120% within 15 min. The changes were transient and after 2 h only one infant had a higher FRC than before surfactant instillation.

In randomized controlled studies using natural surfactants [1, 10], the most immediate response has been an increase in oxygenation. The increase in FRC found in our preliminary studies and also by Edberg et al. [9] and Goldsmith et al. [11] is in agreement with these findings. Changes in dynamic compliance have been less evident during the first 1–24 h after both natural surfactant [6, 7, 11] and artificial surfactant treatment [8]. However, our compliance measurements using the interrupter technique indicate that surfactant instillation does reduce lung retractile force pressure.

We suggest that different surfactant preparations vary in timing, duration and magnitude of effects on lung mechanics. Further studies are needed to evaluate the specific properties of surfactant preparations and their direct or indirect effects on pulmonary mechanics. Presently we are investigating the effects on lung mechanics of high (200 mg/kg) versus low (100 mg/kg) dose of Curosurf. We speculate that future various surfactant preparation may have different indications for use in clinical practice. Indication may differ according to the need for a rapid immediate change in lung function, e.g. with Curosurf or other natural surfactants, or a more gradual change, e.g. with Exosurf or other artificial preparations.

Acknowledgements

This work was supported by grants from the Swedish Medical Research Council (No. 4732), the Medical Faculty, Lund University, and Samariten Research Foundation.

References

1 Collaborative European Multicenter Study Group: Surfactant replacement therapy for severe neonatal respiratory distress syndrome: An international randomized clinical trial. Pediatrics 1988;82:683–691.
2 Jobe A, Ikegami M, Glatz T, Yoshida Y, Diakomanolis E, Padbury J: Duration and characteristics of treatment of premature lambs with natural surfactant. J Clin Invest 1981;67:370–375.
3 Jonmarker C, Castor R, Drefelt B, Werner O: An analyzer for in-line measurement of expiratory sulphur hexafluoride concentration. Anesthesiology 1985;63:84–88.
4 Vilstrup CT, Björklund L, Larsson A, Lachman B, Werner O: FRC and ventilation homogeneity in mechanically ventilated small neonates. J Appl Physiol 1992; in press.
5 Gottfried SB, Rossi A, Calverley PMA, Zocchi L, Millic-Emili J: Interrupter technique for measurement of respiratory mechanics in anesthetized cats. J Appl Physiol 1984;56:681–690.
6 Davis JM, Veness-Meehan K, Notter RH, Bhutani VK, Kendig JW, Shapiro DI: Changes in pulmonary mechanics after the administration of surfactant to infants with respiratory distress syndrome. N Engl J Med 1988;319:476–479.
7 Couser RJ, Ferrara TB, Ebert J, Haekstra RE, Fangman JJ: Effects of exogenous surfactant therapy on dynamic compliance during mechanical breathing in preterm infants with hyaline membrane disease. J Pediatr 1990;116:119–124.
8 Armsby DH, Bellon G, Carlisle K, Rector D, Baldwin R, Stevenson DK, Long WA, Ariagno RL: Two rescue doses of Exosurf improve respiratory system static compliance at one week (abstract). Am Rev Resp Dis 1991;143;A721.
9 Edberg KE, Ekström-Jodal B, Hallman M, Hjalmarsson O, Sandberg K, Silberberg AC: Immediate effects on lung function of instilled human surfactant in mechanically ventilated newborn infants with IRDS. Acta Paediatr Scand 1990;79:750–755.
10 Fujiwara T, Konichi M, Chida S, Okuyama K, Ogawa Y, Takeuchi Y, Nishida H, Kito H, Fujimura M, Nakamura H, Hashimoto T: Surfactant replacement therapy with a single post ventilatory dose of a reconstituted bovine surfactant in preterm neonates with respiratory distress syndrome: Final analyses of a multicenter, double-blind, randomized trial and comparison with similar trials. Pediatrics 1990;86:753–764.
11 Goldsmith LS, Greenspan JS, Rubenstein SD, Wolfson MR, Shaffer TH: Immediate improvement in lung volume after exogenous surfactant: Alveolar recruitment versus increased distention. J Pediatr 1991; 119:424–428.

Original Paper

Biol Neonate 1992;61(suppl 1):48–53

Hervé Walti[a]
Michèle Boulé[b]
Guy Moriette[a]
Jean-Pierre Relier[a]

Service de Médecine Néonatale
[a] Hôpital Port-Royal,
[b] Laboratoire de Physiologie,
Hôpital Trousseau, Paris, France

Pulmonary Functional Outcome at One Year of Age in Infants Treated with Natural Porcine Surfactant at Birth

Key Words
Respiratory distress syndrome
Pulmonary surfactants
Functional residual capacity
Lung compliance

Abstract
This prospective study was designed to assess pulmonary function (functional residual capacity, FRC; dynamic lung compliance, C_{Ldyn}; and total pulmonary resistance, R_L) at 1 year of corrected age in infants with neonatal respiratory distress syndrome treated with natural porcine surfactant (Curosurf) (n = 13), as compared to nontreated control infants (n = 9). Values from 21 healthy infants of similar age served as reference. We found similar pulmonary dysfunction (decreased C_{Ldyn}, elevated R_L) in both patient groups. These results suggest that surfactant replacement therapy does not affect pulmonary function at 1 year of age in infants who survive respiratory distress syndrome.

Introduction

The use of exogenous surfactant for the prevention or treatment of respiratory distress syndrome (RDS) has increased the incidence of survival without bronchopulmonary dysplasia (BPD) [1]. However, up to now the long-term respiratory outcome of babies treated with surfactant has not been well evaluated. The incidence of respiratory symptoms of infants treated at birth with surfactant has been reported to be similar to that in controls [2–9]. Preliminary results of pulmonary function tests performed between 9 and 12 months of age showed no differences between surfactant-treated and control babies [10, 11].

We have previously reported residual abnormalities of pulmonary function in infants [12] and in children [13] who were preterm and treated with mechanical ventilation but not with exogenous surfactant. In the present prospective study we compared pulmonary function at 1 year of corrected age in infants

Dr. Hervé Walti
Service de Médecine Néonatale
Hôpital Port-Royal
123, boulevard de Port-Royal
F–75014 Paris (France)

0006–3126/92/
0617–0048$2.75/0

Table 1. Clinical studies with Curosurf in Port-Royal Hospital 1986–1990

Study design	Total number of cases		Number of survivors		Patients with pulmonary function test at 1 year	
	treated	controls	treated	controls	treated	controls
Single dose[1]	15	15	9	11	6	7
Single vs. multiple doses[2]	7 vs 6	–[3]	4 vs. 4	–[3]	2 vs. 2	–[3]
Early vs. late treatment[4]	12	6	10	6	3	2
Total	40	21	27	17	13	9

1 Data combined from refs. 15 and 17.
2 Data from ref. 18.
3 No nontreated control cases.
4 Data from ref. 19.

treated in the early neonatal period with a natural porcine surfactant with corresponding data from nontreated control infants.

Material and Methods

Characterization of Surfactant

Curosurf is a natural surfactant isolated by chloroform-methanol extraction and liquid-gel chromatography. Derived from minced pig lung, it contains about 99% polar lipids, mainly phospholipids, and 1% low-molecular-weight hydrophobic surfactant-associated proteins (SP-B and SP-C). The preparation and the structural and functional characterization of Curosurf has been fully described elsewhere [14].

Patient Groups

From 1986 to 1990, our institution participated in the Collaborative European Multicenter Study Group which undertook several randomized clinical trials in order to assess the efficacy of Curosurf for the treatment of babies with severe RDS [15–19].

Sixty-one babies were recruited from our neonatal unit in 4 randomized rescue trials (table 1).

Thirty of these babies were enrolled in 2 controlled trials using a single dose of Curosurf [15, 17] with the following common criteria for entry:
(1) Birth weight 700–2,000 g.
(2) Clinical and radiological findings typical of RDS.
(3) Age at treatment 2–15 h.
(4) Need for mechanical ventilation.
(5) Fraction of inspired oxygen (FiO_2) ≥ 0.6.
(6) No complicating disease.

All the treated babies received a single dose of Curosurf (200 mg/kg) instilled into the airways as previously described [15]. No placebo was instilled in control babies.

Thirteen babies were enrolled in the 'single vs. multiple doses' trial of Curosurf with the same criteria for entry as described above [18]. The babies were randomized to be treated either with a single dose of Curosurf (200 mg/kg) or with the same initial dose (200 mg/kg) plus two additional doses of 100 mg/kg 12 and 24 h later if the baby still required $FiO_2 > 0.21$.

Eighteen babies were enrolled in the 'early vs. late treatment' trial [9]. Babies with birth weight 700–2,000 g, age 2–24 h, no complicating disease and RDS requiring mechanical ventilation with FiO_2 0.40–0.59 were randomized to 'early' treatment with a single dose of Curosurf (200 mg/kg) or to 'late' treatment (200 mg/kg) if $FiO_2 \geq 0.6$ was attained in the first 48 h of life.

Forty-four (72%) of the 61 babies enrolled in these trials survived to one year. All survivors were followed-up in our out-patient clinic. We planned to perform pulmonary function testing at 1 year and in this report we present results from 22 infants (50% of those surviving). Thirteen received Curosurf in the neonatal period (treated group), and 9 did not (control group). Some important characteristics of both groups, including FiO_2 and arterial to alveolar PO_2 ratio (a/APO_2) [20] at randomization, ventilator efficiency index

Table 2. Characteristics of patients in the Curosurf-treated, control and reference groups at randomization and pulmonary function testing

Characteristics	Patient groups		
	Curosurf-treated (n = 13)	controls (n = 9)	reference group (n = 21)
Neonatal			
Birth weight, g	1,390 (1,080–1,750)	1,630 (860–1,980)	–
Gestational age, weeks	30 (28–34)	31 (28–32)	–
Age at randomization, h	9 (3–21)	8 (7–18)	–
FiO_2, %	70 (45–100)	60 (50–75)	–
a/A PO_2	0.13 (0.06–0.18)	0.15 (0.09–0.24)	–
VEI	0.13 (0.06–0.18)	0.11 (0.08–0.16)	–
Incidence of BPD	5 (38%)	5 (55%)	–
At pulmonary function testing			
Corrected age, months	12 (10–17)	13 (10–14)	12 (4–14)
Height, cm	75 (67–80)	73 (67–80)	72 (66–80)

There are no statistically significant differences between the groups.

(VEI), an analog of lung compliance [21], and presence of BPD (defined as oxygen dependency at day 28) are listed in table 2. Corrected age and height at the time of pulmonary function test are also given in table 2. No statistically significant differences were found for any of these parameters.

Pulmonary Function Testing

This was performed by one of us (M.B.) who was not aware of the clinical data. The method has been reported in detail before [12, 13]. The infants were tested asleep in the supine position and when necessary, after light sedation with chloral hydrate (< 50 mg/kg). We measured functional residual capacity (FRC) by the helium dilution technique [22] and dynamic lung compliance (C_{Ldyn}) and total pulmonary resistance (R_L) using an oesophageal balloon for transpulmonary pressure measurements [23]. In contrast to our previous studies [12, 13], the patient was connected to the pneumotachygraph by means of a face mask, rather than a mouth piece. PaO_2 and $PaCO_2$ were measured in arterialized capillary blood collected from the ear lobe of awake infants [24]. We compared the results of pulmonary function tests in the two groups with values from 21 healthy infants of similar corrected age and weight previously studied in our laboratory with the same methods (reference group). Our present values of R_L included nasal resistance and cannot be directly compared to the values of R_L obtained in our previous studies.

Statistical Analysis

All the data are given as median (range). Differences between groups were evaluated with non-parametric tests: Mann-Whitney or Kruskal-Wallis. $p < 0.05$ was taken as significant.

Results

FRC

The values were similar in the treated group (207 [137–317] ml), the control group (235 [142–260] ml) and the reference group (215 [147–281] ml) (fig. 1a).

C_{Ldyn}

Values observed in the treated group (12 [7–19] ml/cm H_2O) and in the control group (15 [6–19] ml/cm H_2O) were both lower than those in the reference group (19 [14–21] ml/

cm H_2O) ($p < 0.001$). No statistical difference was demonstrated between the treated and the control group (fig. 1b).

R_L

Values were similar in the treated (34 [30–85] cm $H_2O/l \cdot s$) and the control group (26 [16–56] cm $H_2O/l \cdot s$) (fig. 1c).

PaO_2 and $PaCO_2$

The values of PaO_2 in the treated and control groups were 85 [69–95] and 82 [64–107] mm Hg, respectively (NS). The values of $PaCO_2$ in the treated and control groups were 37 [28–41] and 38 [34–41] mm Hg, respectively (NS). None of the values of PCO_2 and only one value of PaO_2 in the control group were more than 2 SD from the mean of our reference population [24].

Discussion

Pulmonary function was prospectively evaluated at 1 year of corrected age in two groups of infants who survived after severe RDS. One group was treated with a natural porcine surfactant (Curosurf) in the neonatal period and the second group served as controls. We found similar pulmonary dysfunction in both groups, in spite of the improvement in lung function and short-term outcome which had been obtained following treatment with Curosurf in the neonatal period [15–19]. For both groups the observed abnormalities, decreased C_L and elevated R_L, are in agreement with our previous findings in survivors of neonatal RDS who did not receive surfactant [12, 13], and with the results of others [25, 26]. Our results are also in agreement with those of two preliminary studies performed in infants with RDS treated with other surfactants [10, 11]. In the first study [10] pulmonary function tests were

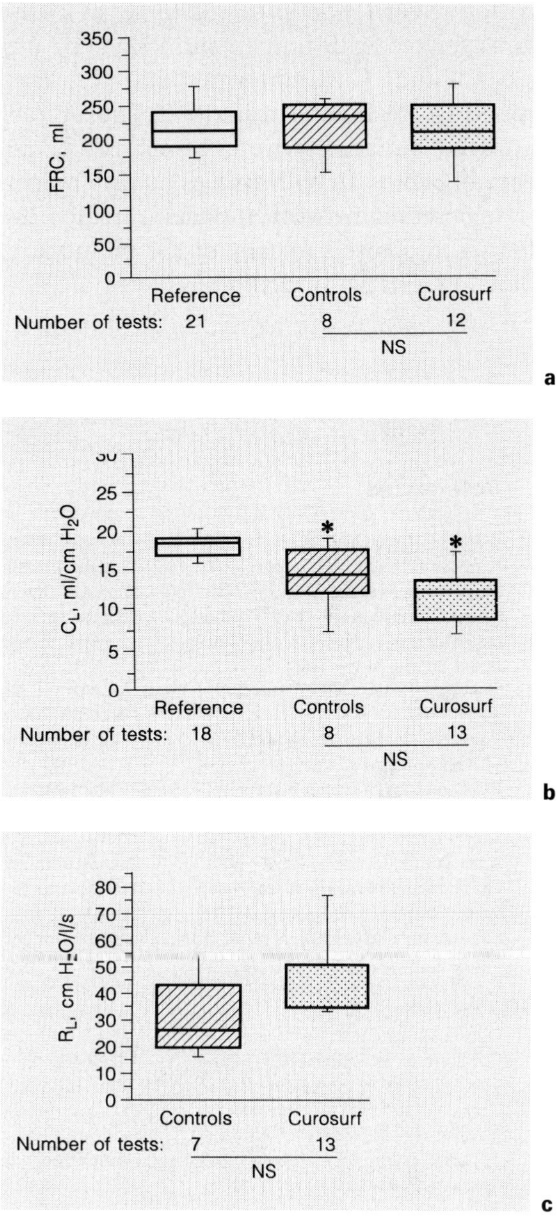

Fig. 1a-c: Results of pulmonary function testing at 1 year of corrected age in Curosurf-treated and control infants. A group of 21 healthy infants of similar age served as a reference group. The top, the bottom and the line in the box represent the 75th, 25th and 50th percentile (median) of the values, respectively. The top and the bottom of the 'moustache' represent the 90th and 10th percentile, respectively. NS = No statistically significant difference. *$p < 0.001$ vs. reference group.

performed at 9 months corrected age in 24 infants treated with human surfactant. In the second study [11], performed at 1 year corrected age, 59 infants treated with Exosurf (an artificial surfactant) were compared to 26 control babies. In both studies no differences were observed between surfactant-treated infants and controls for any of the pulmonary function tests performed.

In conclusion our results, although obtained on a rather small number of patients, suggest that surfactant replacement therapy does not affect pulmonary function at one year of corrected age in infants who survive RDS. However, greater number of babies need to be studied before late long-term effects of surfactant replacement on pulmonary function can be established.

References

1 Walti H, Couchard M, Relier JP: Exogenous surfactant in the management of hyaline membrane disease; in Bourbon JR (ed): Pulmonary Surfactant: Biochemical, Functional, Regulatory, and Clinical Concepts. Boston, CRC Press, 1991, pp 395–429.

2 Vaucher YE, Merritt TA, Hallman M, Jarvenpaa AL, Telsey AM, Jones BL: Neurodevelopmental and respiratory outcome in early childhood after human surfactant treatment. Am J Dis Child 1988;142:927–930.

3 Dunn MS: Intermediate and long term outcome in surfactant treated infants; in Ekelund L, Jonson B, Malm L (eds): Surfactant and the Respiratory Tract. Amsterdam, Elsevier, 1989, pp 207–219.

4 Dunn M, Shennan AT, Hoskins EM, Lennox K, Enhorning G: Two-year follow-up of infants enrolled in a randomized trial of surfactant replacement therapy for prevention of neonatal respiratory distress syndrome. Pediatrics 1988;82:543–547.

5 Jain L, Vidyasagar D, Raju TNK: Developmental outcome of infants from surfactant trials. Pediatr Res 1989;25:255A.

6 Vohr BR, Coll CG, Roberts JD, Brown LJ, Oh W: Decreased morbidities during the first year in very low birth weight (< 1,250 g) infants treated with single dose surfactant TA (STA). Pediatr Res 1989;25:235A.

7 Ware J, Taeusch HW, Soll R, Mc Cormick MC: Health and developmental outcomes of a surfactant controlled trial: Follow up at 2 years. Pediatrics 1990;85:1103–1107.

8 Morley CJ, Morley R: Follow-up of premature babies treated with artificial surfactant (ALEC). Arch Dis Child 1990;65:667–669.

9 Collaborative European Multicenter Study Group: Two year follow-up of babies enrolled in a European multicenter trial of porcine surfactant replacement for severe neonatal respiratory distress syndrome. Eur J Pediatr, in press.

10 Heldt GP, Rosas F, Merritt TA: Pulmonary function of infants treated with human surfactant: Assessment at nine months. Pediatr Res 1989;25:366A.

11 Bhutani VK, Abassi S, Gerdes JS: Long-term pulmonary outcome of infants treated with surfactant for respiratory distress: Exosurf trial. Pediatr Res 1991;29:309A.

12 Moriette G, Gaudebout C, Clement A, Boule M, Bion B, Relier JP, Gaultier C: Pulmonary function at 1 year of age in survivors of neonatal respiratory distress: A multivariate analysis of factors associated with sequelae. Pediatr Pulmonol 1987;3:242–250.

13 Lebourges F, Moriette G, Boule M, Delaperche MF, Relier JP, Gaultier C: Pulmonary function in infancy and in childhood following mechanical ventilation in the neonatal period. Pediatr Pulmonol 1990;9:34–40.

14 Robertson B, Curstedt T, Johanson J, Jörnvall H, Kobayashi T: Structural and functional characterization of porcine surfactant isolated by liquid gel chromatography. Prog Respir Res 1990;25:237–246.

15 Collaborative European Multicenter Study Group: Surfactant replacement therapy for severe neonatal respiratory distress syndrome: An international randomized clinical trial. Pediatrics 1988;82:683–691.

16 Collaborative European Multicenter Study Group: Factors influencing the clinical response to surfactant replacement therapy in babies with severe respiratory distress syndrome. Eur J Pediatr 1991;150:433–439.

17 Walti H, Relier JP, Huon C, Monset-Couchard M, Scemama M, De Gamarra E, Moriette G, Curstedt T, Robertson B: Traitement des formes sévères de la maladie des membranes hyalines par une dose unique d'un surfactant exogéne d'origine porcine. Un essai randomisé: Effets immédiats et devenir à 28 jours de vie. Arch Fr Pédiatr 1990;47:329–334.

18 Speer CP, Robertson B, Curstedt T, Compagnone D, Gefeller O, Harms K, Herting E, Halliday HL, McClure G, Reid M, Tubman R, Herin P, Noack G, Kok J, Koppe J, van Sonderen L, Laufkötter E, Köhler W, Boenich H, Albrecht K, Hanssler L, Haim M, Oetomo SB, Okken A, Altfeld PC, Gronek P, Kachel W, Relier J-P, Walti H: Randomized European multicenter trial of surfactant replacement therapy for severe neonatal respiratory distress syndrome: Single versus multiple doses of Curosurf. Pediatrics 1992;89:13–20.

19 Bevilacqua G, Parmigiani S, Trial Participants: Timing of surfactant therapy for neonatal RDS; in Bevilacqua G, Parmigiani S, Robertson B (eds): Surfactants in Clinical Practice. Chur, Harwood, in press.

20 Gilbert R, Keighley JF: The arterial/alveolar oxygen tension ratio: An index of gas exchange applicable to varying inspired oxygen concentrations. Am Rev Respir Dis 1974;109: 142–145.

21 Kwong MS, Egan AE, Notter RH, Shapiro DL: Double-blind clinical trial of calf lung surfactant extract for the prevention of hyaline membrane disease in extremely premature infants. Pediatrics 1985;76: 585–592.

22 Gaultier C, Boule M, Allaire Y, Clement A, Girard F: Growth of lung volumes during the first three years of life. Bull Eur Physiopathol Respir 1979;15:1103–1116.

23 Gaultier C, Allaire Y, Pappo A, Girard F, Gerbeaux J: Resistance pulmonaire chez l'enfant sain et l'enfant asthmatique: Corrélation avec le VEMS et la compliance pulmonaire dynamique. Rev Fr Mal Respir 1975;3:827–836.

24 Gaultier C, Allaire Y, Clement A, Buvry A, Girard F: Determination of capillary oxygen tension in infants and children. Bull Eur Physiopathol Respir 1978;14:287–297.

25 Lindroth M, Jonson B, Svenningsen NV, Mortensson W: Pulmonary mechanics, chest X-ray and lung disease after mechanical ventilation in low birth weight infants. Acta Paediatr Scand 1980;69:761–770.

26 Gerhardt T, Hehre D, Feller F, Reifenberg L, Bancalari E: Serial determination of pulmonary function in infants with chronic lung disease. J Pediatr 1987;110:448–456.

Original Paper

Biol Neonate 1992;61(suppl 1):54–58

T. Richard J. Tubman[a]
Simon J. Rankin[b]
Henry L. Halliday[a, b]
Stewart S. Johnston[b]

[a] Neonatal Intensive Care Unit, Royal Maternity Hospital, Belfast,
[b] Department of Ophthalmology,
[c] Department of Child Health, The Queen's University of Belfast, UK

Surfactant Replacement Therapy and the Prevalence of Acute Retinopathy of Prematurity

Key Words

Respiratory distress syndrome
Pulmonary surfactants
Retinopathy of prematurity

Abstract

To determine if surfactant replacement treatment is associated with an increase in the prevalence of retinopathy of prematurity (ROP) we studied 76 preterm babies who were treated with porcine surfactant (Curosurf) for severe respiratory distress syndrome from 1985 to 1990. Babies were first examined by indirect ophthalmoscopy at the equivalent of 32 weeks post-menstrual age and subsequently at 2-week intervals until discharge from hospital. Findings were documented according to the International Classification of ROP. Sixty-two (82%) babies survived to discharge, 7 survivors were not examined due to transfer elsewhere. Acute ROP developed in 14 (29%) of the 49 babies examined (7 stage I, 4 stage II, 2 stage III, and 1 stage IV); one baby required cryotherapy. No baby of birthweight > 1,500 g developed ROP. The prevalence of ROP was similar to that reported for non-surfactant-treated very-low-birthweight babies. We conclude that Curosurf treatment does not increase the risk of acute ROP in surviving very-low-birthweight babies.

Introduction

Acute proliferative retinopathy of prematurity (ROP) remains a problem of the preterm, very-low-birthweight baby despite, and to some extent due to, advances in neonatal intensive care. The prevalence and severity of ROP are greatest in babies of < 1,500 g birthweight or < 31 weeks of gestational age. Hyperoxaemia has been implicated in the genesis of ROP [1], but other factors including low gestational age, acidosis and hypercarbia are

Dr. Richard Tubman
Neonatal Intensive Care Unit
Birmingham Maternity Hospital
Edgbaston
Birmingham B15 (UK)

0006–3126/92/
0617–0054$2.75/0

also involved [2]. Thus, the smallest sickest babies are at greatest risk of developing ROP.

Surfactant replacement therapy has become an established treatment for respiratory distress syndrome (RDS). Administration of natural surfactant produces an acute increase in PaO_2 in the majority of babies; in the Collaborative European Multicenter Trial of porcine surfactant (Curosurf) replacement, a dramatic rise in mean PaO_2 was seen within 5 min of treatment, reaching levels of almost 20 kPa [3]. In addition to these acute improvements in oxygenation, surfactant has been shown to reduce mortality and the incidence of major complications, particularly air leaks [3, 4]. Thus, these babies survive but often require prolonged periods of intensive care and they may develop other complications such as patent ductus arteriosus, intraventricular haemorrhage or septicaemia.

It is possible that use of surfactant might increase the risk of ROP, given the rapid surges in PaO_2, and the increased survival of sick tiny babies [5]. We have studied the prevalence of acute ROP in a group of Curosurf-treated babies managed in the Royal Maternity Hospital, Belfast, over a 5-year period.

Material and Methods

The babies studied included those enrolled in a number of European multicentre trials of surfactant replacement, and those treated openly between trials, in the period 1985–1990. Babies with clinical and radiological evidence of RDS, who were being mechanically ventilated with a median (range) fraction of inspired oxygen of 0.80 (0.4–1.0), were treated with Curosurf at a median (range) of 5 (2–31) h from birth. Curosurf was instilled intratracheally in 2 aliquots each followed by 1 min of manual ventilation, before reconnection to the ventilator.

Babies were examined by one consultant paediatric ophthalmologist. Phenylephrine 2.5% and cyclopentolate 1% eye drops were instilled to produce pupillary dilatation 30 min before indirect ophthalmoscopy, which was carried out at the cotside. The initial examination was performed at the equivalent of 32 weeks post-menstrual age and repeated every 2 weeks until 36 weeks post-menstrual age or regression of eye signs whichever was sooner. If ROP was found, examination was repeated weekly unless stage II + or greater was present, in which case examination was performed more frequently. A number of babies were followed-up after discharge from hospital.

We staged ROP according to the 1984 International Classification [6], i.e. stage I, a demarcation line between avascular and vascularised retina; stage 2, ridge formation; stage 3, a ridge with extraretinal fibrovascular proliferation, and stage 4, retinal detachment. The presence of 'plus' disease, that is increasing dilatation and tortuosity of the peripheral retinal vessels, was also recorded.

Results

Seventy-six preterm babies were treated with Curosurf in the period 1985–1990. There were 45 boys and 31 girls. Sixty-six (87%) of these were <1,500 g birthweight and 33 (43%) <1,000 g. Mean (SD) birthweight was 1,095 (312) g and gestational age 27.6 (2.0) weeks. Sixty-one (80%) babies received a single dose of Curosurf, equivalent to 100–200 mg/kg of phospholipid depending on the trial in which they were entered; the remainder received up to two additional doses of 100 mg/kg within 24 h of the first dose.

Figure 1 shows changes in mean arterial/alveolar oxygen tension ratio (a/APO_2) to 24 h after surfactant replacement. There was a rapid, almost 3-fold sustained rise in mean a/APO_2 from 0.1 pretreatment to 0.32 at 1 h after treatment. This improvement persisted for at least 48 h. Table 1 shows morbidity and mortality rates; of the 76 babies treated, 62 (82%) survived to discharge from hospital.

Not all of the babies could be examined ophthalmologically in our unit due to transfer of some to other hospitals before 32 weeks post-menstrual age. Six of the 9 babies with

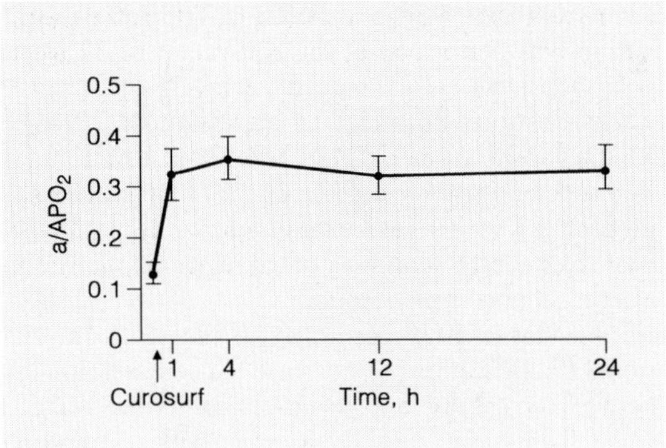

Fig. 1. Changes in arterial/alveolar oxygen tension ratio (a/APO_2, mean ± 95% confidence intervals) before and in the first 24 h after Curosurf treatment (arrow).

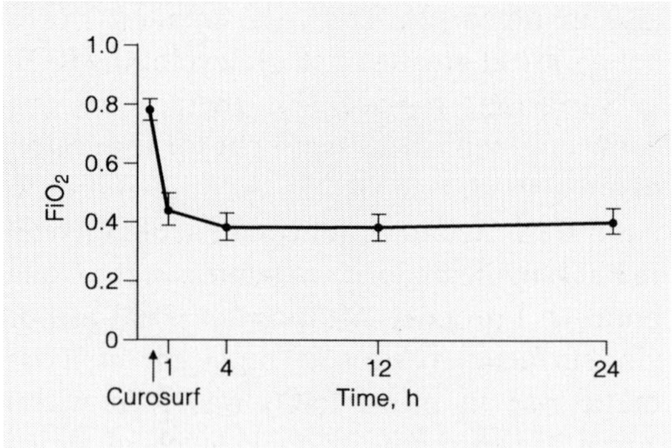

Fig. 2. Changes in fraction of inspired oxygen concentration (FiO_2, mean ± 95% confidence intervals) before and in the first 24 h after Curosurf treatment (arrow).

Table 1. Morbidity and mortality in Curosurf-treated babies (n = 76)

Complications	n	%
Patent ductus arteriosus	30	39
Pneumothorax	21	28
Intraventricular haemorrhage (grade III/IV)	20	26
Bronchopulmonary dysplasia	33	43
Survival to discharge	62	82

Table 2. Prevalence of acute ROP by stage in survivors < 1,500 g birthweight (n = 49)

Stage of ROP	n	%
I	7	14
II	2	4
II+	2	4
III	2	4
IV	1	2
Total	14	29

birthweight ≥ 1,500 g were available for examination and none developed ROP. Forty-nine of the 53 surviving babies < 1,500 g were examined; of these 14 (29%) had signs of ROP. Of the 22 survivors weighing < 1,000 g at birth, 8 (36%) had ROP. Table 2 shows the prevalence of acute ROP by stage in very-low-birthweight survivors who were examined. Two infants developed stage 3 disease, but did not reach threshold for cryotherapy; one of these died of bronchopulmonary dysplasia in hospital at the age of 200 days, whilst the other's eye signs regressed completely. One baby progressed to retinal detachment after discharge from hospital despite cryotherapy and he subsequently died from sudden infant death syndrome. All seven infants who developed stage II ROP or greater were born at 25–26 weeks of gestation and all developed other complications including intraventricular haemorrhage (n = 7), periventricular leukomalacia (n = 2), septicaemia (n = 7), patent ductus arteriosus (n = 2), seizures (n = 3), and bronchopulmonary dysplasia (defined as persistent oxygen requirement at 28 d with typical radiologial features) (n = 6).

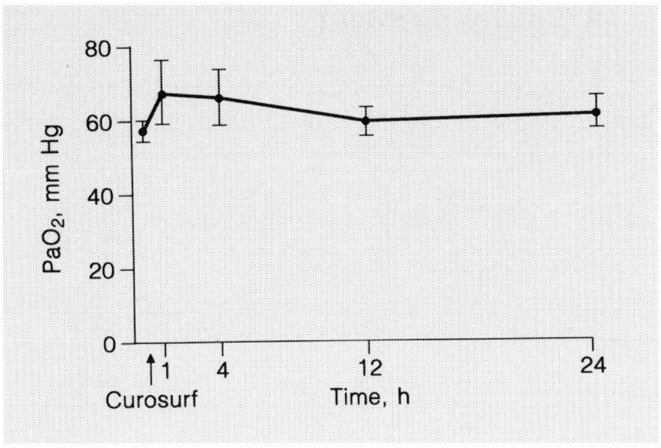

Fig. 3. Changes in PaO_2 (mm Hg, mean ± 95% confidence intervals) before and in the first 24 h after Curosurf treatment (arrow).

Discussion

RDS is a common problem in preterm babies, developing in 65% of babies <1,500 g birthweight and in 80% of those <1,000 g [7]. In these babies hypo- and hyperoxemia, hypercarbia, respiratory and metabolic acidosis are frequently encountered and all of these factors have been shown to be significantly associated with the development of acute ROP [2, 8]. Progression of ROP to advanced disease appears to be determined by the severity of the early insult to the immature retina [2]. Estimates of the prevalence of ROP range from 3–5% [9] to 49% [10]. This wide range can be partially accounted for both by differing examination protocols and variable survival rates between units. Surfactant replacement has been a significant advance in neonatal care in the past decade, but recently concern has been voiced that the improved survival and sometimes prolonged oxygen dependence due to this new therapy might put immature babies at a greater risk of developing ROP [5].

Our study was not controlled as the highly significant reduction in mortality due to surfactant replacement would make such a study unethical to perform. We have no reliable historical data from the pre-surfactant era in Belfast (before 1985), as the diagnosis and classification of ROP was not uniform prior to the introducton of the International Classification in 1984.

However, our results can be compared with those from other units. Prendiville and Schulenburg [2] prospectively studied the prevalence of ROP in a group of 140 infants who had a similar mean birthweight and gestational age, and similar survival rates to our babies, but who did not receive surfactant therapy. They found an almost identical overall prevalence of ROP in babies <1,500 g (30 vs. 29%), but a greater prevalence of severe (stage 3 and 4) ROP (11 vs. 6%). ROP in babies less than 1,000 g was also more frequent than in our study (50 vs. 36%). The most severe stages of ROP occurred in the smallest, illest babies. A number of reasons other than chance may be postulated as to why we found fewer cases of severe ROP. Firstly, since the conclusion of the Collaborative European Multicenter Trial in 1987 [3], it has been our practice to rapidly reduce the fraction of inspired oxygen following Curosurf administration using continuous recording of oxygen saturation by pulse oximetry (fig. 2). Secondly, our babies were enrolled in trials whose protocols demanded close attention to blood gas values and blood pressure, thereby allowing prompt correction of any deleterious changes. Figure 3 shows how fluctuations in PaO_2 were kept to a minimum. These measures may have helped reduce the severity of any early insults on the developing retina.

In conclusion, we have not found an increase in the prevalence of proliferative retinopathy of prematurity occurring as a result of the introduction of surfactant replacement. This is encouraging, but since increasing numbers of very immature babies are now surviving, we must continue to closely monitor them for signs of retinopathy of prematurity.

Acknowledgement

We should like to acknowledge the secretarial assistance in Miss Samantha Lane in the preparation of the manuscript.

References

1 Silverman WA: Retrolentral Fibroplasia: A Modern Parable. New York, Grune & Stratton, 1980.
2 Prendiville A, Schulenburg WE: Clinical factors associated with retinopathy of prematurity. Arch Dis Child 1988;63:522–527.
3 Collaborative European Multicenter Study Group: Surfactant replacement therapy for severe neonatal repsiratory distress syndrome: An international randomized clinical trial. Pediatrics 1988;82:683–691.
4 Morley CJ: Surfactant treatment for premature babies. A review of clinical trials. Arch Dis Child 1991;66: 445–450.
5 Kalina RE: Treatment of retinal detachment due to retinopathy of prematurity: Documented disappointment. Ophthalmology 1981;98:3–4.
6 Committee for the Classification of Retinopathy of Prematurity: An international classification of retinopathy of prematurity. Pediatrics 1984;74:127–133.
7 McClure BG, Halliday HL: Respiratory distress syndrome; in McClure BG, Halliday HL, Thompson W (eds): Perinatal Medicine. London, Baillière Tindall, 1988, pp 76–93.
8 Avery GB, Glass P: Retinopathy of prematurity: What causes it? Clin Perinatol 1988;15:917–928.
9 Yu VYH, Hookham DN, Nave JRM: Retrolental fibroplasia. A controlled study of four years experience in an neonatal intensive care unit. Arch Dis Child 1982;57:247–252.
10 Ng YK, Fielder AR, Shaw DE, Levene MI: Epidemiology of retinopathy of prematurity. Lancet 1988;ii: 1235–1238.

Original Paper

Biol Neonate 1992;61(suppl 1):59–65

Johannes Egberts

Department of Obstetrics and Gynecology, University of Leiden, The Netherlands

Estimated Costs of Different Treatments of the Respiratory Distress Syndrome in a Large Cohort of Preterm Infants of Less than 30 Weeks of Gestation

Key Words

Respiratory distress syndrome
Infant, premature
Corticosteroids
Costs and cost analysis
Pulmonary surfactants
Length of stay

Abstract

Within a model cohort of 1,000 preterm infants of < 30 weeks of gestation, the incidence and mortality of RDS change if corticosteroids are used prenatally and surfactant prophylactically or therapeutically after birth. Combined pre- and postnatal therapies give the best results: approximately 125 extra survivors. Therapeutic surfactant administration even in combination with prenatal corticosteroids has cost implications because extra intensive care beds (7–11%) are needed. More special care places (12–24%) are required after each type of intervention. The estimated costs per extra survivor are the lowest for prenatal corticosteroid administration. The combination of corticosteroids prenatally and prophylactic surfactant postnatally seems to be most cost-effective because it produces the greatest number of survivors and the lowest number of intensive and high dependency care days in hospital.

Introduction

Prenatal administration of glucocorticosteroids to pregnant women reduces both mortality and the morbidity due to the respiratory distress syndrome (RDS) in preterm infants [1]. However, these corticosteroids are not always used either because of reticence shown by the obstetricians [2, 3] or the short period between admission to the hospital and the birth of the preterm baby.

In those cases, when corticosteroids are either not given or are ineffective, it is important to have surfactant treatment available. Surfactant treatment to the preterm newborn also reduces morbidity and mortality caused by RDS. In the overviews of the clinical trials [4], odds ratios for mortality and morbidity

Dr. J. Egberts
Department of Obstetrics and Gynecology
University of Leiden
PO Box 9600
NL–2300 RC Leiden (The Netherlands)

0006–3126/92/
0617–0059$2.75/0

are similar whether surfactant is given prophylactically or therapeutically. However, it has been established that prophylaxis will reduce the occurrence of RDS [4].

It has often been suggested, but without evidence, that prophylactic administration of surfactant increases the costs of neonatal care compared to the use of surfactant to treat established RDS. Recent publications from the United Kingdom, United States and Canada have examined the costs of surfactant treatments [5–8]. Differences between the populations of babies studied and health care costs in the various countries may account for the disparity of results.

In this study, data from a well-defined population of preterm infants were used for the calculation of the costs of various types of treatment to prevent or alleviate RDS in preterm neonates.

Materials and Methods

Patients

A population of 468 preterm babies of gestational age < 30 weeks was selected from the 'POPS' (Project on Preterm and Small for gestational age infants) study [9] which describes extensively the obstetric and neonatal findings of all live-born preterm infants in 1983 in the Netherlands. Corticosteroids were not given before birth in this selected population. Of these 468 infants, 309 (= 66 %) developed RDS, of whom 159 (= 51 %) babies died; 65 of the 155 infants, who did not develop RDS, died of other causes.

Effects of Therapy

Estimates of the effects of corticosteroids or surfactant on the incidence of RDS and the mortality due to RDS were derived from overviews and were expressed as typical odds ratios with their 95 % confidence limits (table 1). The typical odds ratios were calculated from corticosteroid trials, reported in the literature involving pregnancies < 31 weeks [1] and from surfactant trials of babies < 30 weeks of gestation [4]. It was assumed that a prenatal administration of corticosteroids for a period long enough of being effective is possible in 75 % of the cases. This treatment is not always possible because corticosteroids cannot be given in all cases of preterm birth. The estimate of the effect of prophylactic surfactant treatment on the incidence of RDS was derived only from those studies in which the results concerning the number of RDS patients were reported [4]. The impacts of the different interventions on the incidence of RDS and mortality was calculated according to the formula of Mugford et al. [5]:

$$Re = [N \cdot Ro \cdot T/(N - Ro)]/[1 + (Ro \cdot T/(N - Ro))]$$

where Re = the expected number with the outcome RDS or death after the intervention, N = total number of babies, Ro = the observed number of babies with the outcome RDS or death without treatment, and T = the typical odds ratio for the effect of the therapy. The odds ratios for the combined treatment with corticosteroids and surfactant were calculated from the number that would be expected after the corticosteroid application alone.

It was assumed that a maximum of 5% of the infants not developing RDS after the intervention, will die from other causes. This correction increases the mortality of the babies without RDS. All calculations were normalized for a cohort of 1,000 babies.

Period of Hospitalization

The definitions of special care and of intensive care and high dependency care are similar to those used in the UK (special care and intensive care levels I and II) [7, 10]. The total mean period of hospitalization for surviving infants of less than 30 weeks of gestation is 79.5 days for infants without RDS and 89.6 days for infants with RDS [9]. The Dutch Society for Pediatrics (Nederlandse Vereniging voor Kindergeneeskunde) estimated in 1987 a mean period of 30 intensive and high depending care days [11] and recalculation leads to 24 intensive and high dependency care days for the surviving infants without RDS and 34 days for those infants with RDS. The period of special care was the same for both groups of infants: 55–56 days. The days of hospitalization, mainly for intensive and high dependency care in infants who died was 3.3 days for babies without RDS and 9.1 days for the infants with RDS [9].

Daily Costs

These are care-related and the price per day is based on the year-price per bed reported in 1990 by the Central Organization for Tariffs of Health Care in the Netherlands, and then corrected for an 80 % occupancy. The re-calculated price for intensive and high dependency care for 1990 was Dfl 1,164 and for special care approximately Dfl 510 per day (US $ 1 = Dfl 1.85).

Table 1. The effect of prenatal administration of corticosteroids and/or postnatal surfactant treatment on the incidence and mortality of RDS in infants < 30 weeks of gestation

Extra intervention	Typical odds ratios (+ 95 % confidence limits)		Incidence figures corrected for 1,000 patients			
	RDS	mortality	RDS		mortality	
			+	–	+RDS	-RDS
None	1	1	660	340	331	139
Corticosteroids	0.38 (0.24–0.60)	0.59 (0.47–0.75)	484	516	267	142
Prophylactic surfactant	0.44 (0.32–0-61)	0.56 (0.43–0.74)	461	539	238	144
Therapeutic surfactant	1	0.60 (0.49–0.75)	660	340	249	139
Corticosteroids +						
Prophylactic surfactant	0.21 (0.11–0.41)	0.42 (0.31–0.62)	292	708	198	146
Therapeutic surfactant	0.48 (0.35–0.68)	0.45 (0.35–0.63)	484	516	206	142

The typical odds ratios for the 'corticosteroid + surfactant' combinations are calculated using the altered numbers for RDS and mortality after the corticosteroid intervention alone.

Costs of Therapy

Prenatal glucocorticosteroid therapy costs approximately Dfl 25, whereas the price of surfactant ranges between Dfl 750 and Dfl 1,500 (a price of Dfl 1,000 is used in the calculations.) It is likely that the number of doses of surfactant will be lower after prophylactic administration than after therapeutical use [12]. Thus, 1.5 and 2.5 doses were used in the calculations for the prophylactic or therapeutic groups, respectively.

Results

Effect of Therapy

The effect of the different types of therapy on the number of RDS patients are shown in table 1. After prenatal corticosteroid treatment the number of babies with RDS would be reduced from 660 to 484 and to 461 after prophylactic administration of surfactant. Although the typical odds ratio for the effect of corticosteroids is lower than that of prophylactic surfactant treatment, the effect is smaller, because of the assumption that a corticosteroid treatment is only possible in 75 % of the cases. The combination of corticosteroids and prophylactic surfactant reduces the number of RDS patients even further to 292. The therapeutic administration of surfactant does not influence the number of babies with RDS (n = 660) and for the combined treatment of corticosteroids + therapeutic surfactant the estimated incidence of RDS is the same as for the corticosteroid therapy alone. The effect of corticosteroids on the reduction of mortality from RDS (n = 267) depends on the percentage of prenatally treated infants and is thus less than that of surfactant. The reduction of mortality is somewhat better if surfactant is given prophylactically instead of therapeutically (238 vs. 249). The mortality decreased further if corticosteroids are given to the mother before birth and surfactant to the newborn afterwards (198 vs. 206). The mortality of babies without RDS increases after most interventions because of a 5% correction factor for the extra survivors with RDS (see 'methods'). The greatest number of extra

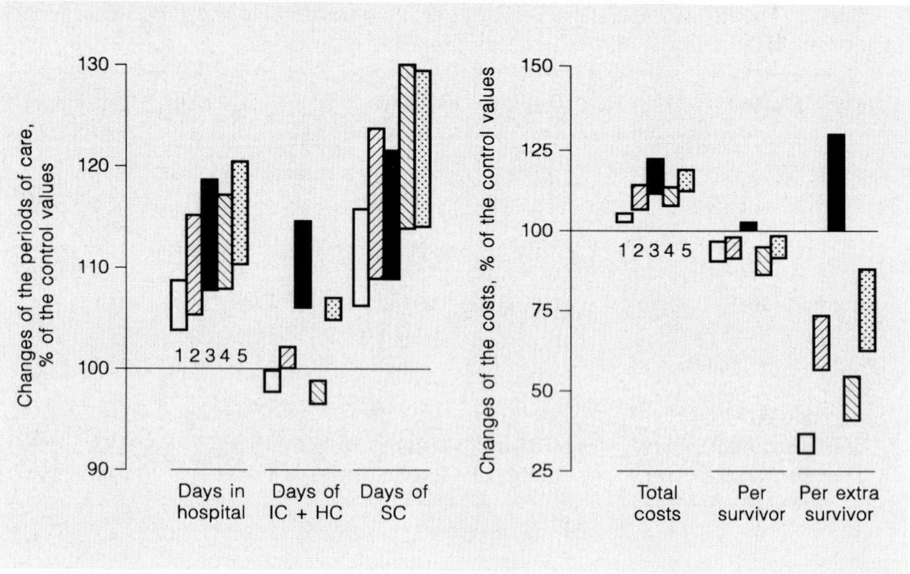

Fig. 1. Estimated changes in the duration of care and of costs after (1) prenatal corticosteroids; (2) prophylactic treatment with surfactant; (3) therapeutic administration of surfactant; (4) corticosteroids + prophylactic surfactant; (5) corticosteroids + therapeutic surfactant. The bars show the 95% confidence limits for each type of intervention.

survivors (n = 126) was found after prenatal corticosteroids and prophylactic surfactant treatment.

Days in Hospital and Their Costs

The total number of days of hospitalization decreases if the number of RDS patients decreases. On the other hand, it increases if more infants survive. The net results of these two effects, in relation to the type of interventions are presented in table 2 and figure 1 shows the 95% conficence limits of changes in the periods of care after different types of intervention. These results are presented as percentages of control values. Each type of intervention requires extra days of hospitalization, increasing the mean period from almost 49 to 57 days after the combined interventions of corticosteroids and therapeutic surfactant. More days of special care (112–124% of the control value) are required after each type of intervention. More intensive and high dependency care days (107–111% of the control value) are needed only if surfactant is given therapeutically. This holds also for the combination of therapeutic surfactant and prenatal corticosteroids. Table 2 shows that the total costs also increase after each type of treatment and figure 1 shows the 95% confidence limits of all these changes. Corticosteroid therapy is less expensive; the total cost increases from Dfl. 37.7 to 39.2 million. The calculations show clearly that costs are higher after surfactant therapy for RDS than after prophylactic surfactant application. Each type of intervention, except for therapeutic surfactant, reduces the cost per survivor, e.g. from Dfl 71.2 to 66.3 thousand after corticosteroids. In comparison with the normal costs per survivor, the costs per extra survivor in-

Table 2. Days in hospital and costs for 1,000 infants of < 30 weeks gestation after prenatal administration of corticosteroids and/or postnatal surfactant treatment

Extra intervention	Days in hospital (× 1,000)			Total costs (× Dfl 1,000,000)	Costs (× Dfl 1,000)	
	total	IC + HC	SC		per survivor	per extra survivor
None	48.9	19.5	29.4	37.7	71.2	(71.2)
Corticosteroids	52.1	19.3	32.8	39.2	66.3	24.3
Prophylactic surfactant	54.0	19.7	34.3	41.6	67.3	43.9
Therapeutic surfactant	55.5	21.5	34.0	44.1	72.0	77.5
Corticosteroids +						
Prophylactic surfactant	55.4	19.0	36.4	41.8	63.7	32.0
Therapeutic surfactant	57.0	20.8	36.2	43.9	67.7	50.8

The results from table 1 are used for the calculation of the number of days of hospitalization and for the calculation of the costs (1 US $ = Dfl 1.85). IC = Intensive care; HC = high dependency care; SC = special care.

crease if surfactant is given therapeutically. The lowest costs per extra survivor (Dfl 24,317) are found after prenatal corticosteroid administration. The effect of corticosteroid treatment also accounts for the relatively low costs per extra survivor after the combined therapies.

Discussion

The present study based on a large population of preterm babies, using typical odds ratios derived from randomized controlled trials [1, 4], should provide reliable estimates of the effects of various treatments in the Netherlands. The estimates may differ from results obtained from other studies based on populations from selected hospitals [5–8].

The calculations within the model show that each type of intervention reduces the neonatal mortality from RDS and, with the exception of the group in which surfactant was given therapeutically, also reduces the incidence of RDS. Farrell et al. [13] had better results after using a combination of corticosteroids and surfactant than after surfactant treatment alone. Their conclusion is supported by our calculations and those of Mugford et al. [5], which strengthen the argument for the use of prenatal corticosteroids whenever possible [2, 3].

The results of the calculations are based on data from 1983 [9], which may no longer be applicable today. A more recent study as accurate as POPS is not available, but a report of the Dutch Health Council (Gezondheidsraad) [11] has presented new estimates for the numbers of preterm infants of < 30 weeks of gestation and born in 1989. These have increased from 562 in 1983 (of which 468 were born without prenatal corticosteroid applications) to approximately 860, partly because of an increase in preterm multiple births, following in vitro fertilization and other forms of assisted reproduction. In comparison with the 468 infants of 1983, the incidence of RDS has decreased by approximately 10% in 1989 and the mortality rate has decreased by approximatley 15–20% [unpubl. results, Working Group Neonatal Pulmonology, Dutch Society of Pediatrics]. The assumption is made that prenatal corticosteroid therapy was given in about 30% of the preterm births in 1989 instead of 17% in 1983. These changes affect the results of the calculations. Given the restriction of the estimate of the 1989 results, and taking into account the effect of the increased number of survivors, the total costs and the total number of days for each level of care are 15–20% higher than those for the POPS population. However, after most interventions, the cost per survivor or per extra survivor differ about 10% between 1989 and 1983. With the exception for the costs after the use of prenatal corticosteroids, the change of costs per extra survivor between 1983 and 1989 is within the 95% conficence limits of the results shown in figure 1. Thus, it may be concluded that the cost analysis, based on data of the POPS study, is still valid.

Different systems of reimbursement between countries make it difficult to compare the results of cost-benefit studies. Nevertheless, the costs per survivor in The Netherlands are between those calculated for neonates in the UK and for those in the USA and Canada [5–8]. The estimate of the Dutch costs was based on the system of fixed daily prices for two levels of care and on the prices of the drugs. Thus, the total costs for treatment are determined mainly by the number of days of hospitalization. The calculations for each type of intervention show that the number of special-care days increases concurrently with the increase in the number of survivors. Furthermore, within the 95% confidence limits, more intensive care beds are required if surfactant is given therapeutically instead of prophylactically. Consequently, prophylactic and not therapeutic surfactant therapy offers to be more cost-effective. Prenatal administration of corticosteroids results in the lowest costs per extra survivor. Although this treatment is the most cost-effective, the combination of corticosteroids and prophylactic surfactant gives a greater number of extra survivors.

The estimates of the costs do not take into account the significant changes in morbidity [1, 4]. These changes will only modify the costs in the Netherlands if they reduce the duration of intensive and high dependency care. Some of these changes reduce the ancillary costs [5, 6, 8], whereas others increase costs because some very preterm infants survive [7] or die later than expected [6]. It is not clear at present how costs change when differences in morbidity occur after prophylactic compared to therapeutic administration of surfactant [8, 12, 14–16].

In this study, the incidence of RDS was 66%. This percentage will decrease if corticosteroids are used more widely. The costs after prophylactic surfactant treatment may then approach those of surfactant used therapeutically. This will occur if too many infants receive expensive surfactant prophylactically without needing it. Such a situation arises when the incidence of RDS ranges between 20 and 25%. This low percentage of babies with RDS is obtained if the upper limit of the gestational age becomes greater than 30 weeks. Although economic considerations indicate that prophylactic administration of surfactant, in combination with prenatal corticosteroids, is a very useful and cost-effective intervention for preventing RDS, ethical arguments make it difficult to give surfactant to approximately 80% of infants who do not need it. However, compromises are possible. Kendig et al. [12] proposed the prophylactic administration of surfactant to all infants born after a pregnancy of less than 27 weeks, because these infants are at a high risk for developing RDS. Another possibility is to give surfactant only when needed and as early as possible before moderate or severe RDS develops. The effects of early intervention are now being studied by several groups and costs may approach those of the best cost-effective procedure, namely prenatal maternal corticosteroid treatment + prophylactic administration of surfactant.

Acknowledgments

I thank Dr. M.J.N.C. Keirse for overviews of surfactant trials from the Oxford Database of Perinatal Trials, and Dr. S.P. Verloove-Vanhorick for her critical remarks and data from the POPS study. The study was partly supported by Praeventiefonds no. 28–1559.

References

1 Crowley P, Chalmers I, Keirse MJNC: The effect of corticosteroid administration before preterm delivery: An overview of the evidence from controlled trials. Br J Obstet Gynaecol 1990;97:11–25.

2 Avery ME: The argument for prenatal administration of dexamethasone to prevent respiratory distress syndrome. J Pediatr 1984;104:240.

3 Neonatal Intensive Care for Low Birthweight Infants: Health Technology Case Study 38. Washington, US Congress, Office of Technology Assessment, 1987.

4a–d Soll RF (ed): (a) Overview 5206; Natural Surfactant Extract Treatment of RDS. (b) Overview 5207; Prophylactic Administration of Natural Surfactant Extract. (c) Overview 5252; Synthetic Surfactant Treatment of RDS. (d) Overview 5253; Prophylactic Administration of Synthetic Surfactant. Oxford, Oxford Database of Perinatal Trials, 1991.

5 Mugford M, Piercy J, Chalmers I: Cost implications of different approaches to the prevention of respiratory distress syndrome. Arch Dis Childh 1991;66:757–764.

6 Maniscalco WM, Kendig JW, Shapiro DL: Surfactant replacement therapy: Impact on hospital charges for premature infants with respiratory distress syndrome. Pediatrics 1989;83:1–6.

7 Tubman TRJ, Halliday HL, Normand C: Cost of surfactant replacement treatment for severe neonatal respiratory distress syndrome: a randomised controlled trial. Br Med J 1990;301:842–845.

8 Shennan A, Dunn M, Possmayer F: Cost-effectiveness of single dose surfactant prophylaxis in infants of less than 30 weeks' gestation. Pediatr Res 1989;25:231A.

9 Verloove-VanHorick SP, Verwey RA: Project on preterm and small for gestational age infants in the Netherlands 1983, Thesis, Leiden University, 1987.

10 British Paediatric Association and British Association for Perinatal Paediatrics: Categories of babies requiring neonatal care. Arch Dis Childh 1984;60:599–600.

11 Intensive Care voor Pasgeborenen: Een behoefteraming. Commissie Intensive Care Neonatologie. Gezondheidsraad, report 1991/6. Den Haag, 1991.

12 Kendig JW, Notter RH, Cox C, Reubens LJ, Davis JM, Maniscalco WM, Sinkin RA, Bartoletti A, Dweck HS, Horgan MJ, Risemberg J, Phalps DL, Shapiro DL: A comparison of surfactant as immediate prophylaxis and as rescue therapy in newborns of less than 30 weeks' gestation. N Engl J Med 1991;324:865–871.

13 Farrell EE, Siver RK, Kimberlin LV, Wolf ES, Dusik JM: Impact of antenatal dexamethasone administration on respiratory distress syndrome in surfactant-treated infants. Am J Obstet Gynecol 1989;161:628–633.

14 Dunn M, Shennan A, Possmayer F: Bovine surfactant replacement therapy in infants less than 30 week's gestation. A randomized trial of prophylaxis vs treatment. Pediatr Res 1990;27:204A.

15 Merritt TA, Hallman M, Berry C, Pohjavuori M, Edwards DK, Jaskelainen J, Grafe MR, Vaucher Y, Wozniak P, Heldt G, Rapola J: Randomized, placebo-controlled trial of human surfactant given a birth versus rescue administration in very low birth weight infants with lung immaturity. J Pediatr 1991;118:581–595.

16 Egberts J, de Winter P, van Bel F: Surfactant prophylaxis in the delivery room; in Bevilacqua G, Parmigiani S, Robertson B (eds): Surfactant in Clinical Practice. Harwood, Chur, 1992, pp 113–119.

Author Index

Subject Index